a novel in cartoons

The
DEMENTIA
Diaries

BY

Matthew Snyman

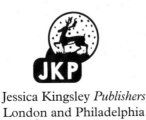

JKP

Jessica Kingsley *Publishers*
London and Philadelphia

First published in 2016
by Jessica Kingsley Publishers
73 Collier Street
London N1 9BE, UK
and
400 Market Street, Suite 400
Philadelphia, PA 19106, USA

www.jkp.com

Library of Congress Cataloging in Publication Data
A CIP catalog record for this book is available from the Library of Congress

British Library Cataloguing in Publication Data
A CIP catalogue record for this book is available from the British Library

ISBN 978 1 78592 032 5
eISBN 978 1 78450 285 0

Printed and Bound in China

TABLE OF CONTENTS

Chapter One "I guess sometimes it's just easier to write it down": Meet Brie, Fred, Sarah and Sam

Chapter Two "Nanny's Braincells": The first signs of dementia

Chapter Three "Puzzled": Ways of coping with dementia

Chapter Four "Shirt, jumper, shirt, jumper, shirt, jumper, cardigan": Things change as dementia progresses

Chapter Five "Mr Table Dancer": Although it can be, dementia's not always a scary thing

Chapter Six "The Christmas Decision": Thinking about the future

THANKS TO...

Emma, Matthew, Vicky, Demetria, KCC,
SILK, DementiaUK, Tom and Pauline, Louie,
Margaret, Harrison, Victoria, Louise, Raisa,
Lorraine, Brian, Cory, Jack, Kyle, Nancy,
Madeline, Imogen, Jasmine, Jack,
FACES of Kent Young Carers,
Matt, Katie and Joshua from MidKent College,
Wendy, Daren from the Beaney, Neville,
East Kent Independent Dementia Support (E.K.I.D.s),
Sue, Alistair, Hilda, Jens Peter, Berit, Georgina, Nicki K,
Tommy on Tour, Keith Oliver, Kiran Rao, Merevale House,
Dementia Friendly Kent Reference Group,
NHS England, Journal of Dementia Care

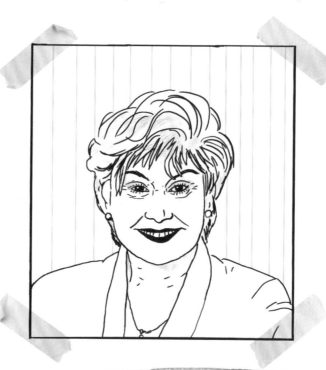

Foreword by
ANGELA RIPPON OBE

The Dementia Diaries are a delight – and a revelation.
The thoughts of these young people coming to terms
with the effect that dementia has on much-loved
members of their families are humorous, humbling and
overlaid with uncompromising honesty.

They demonstrate a remarkably mature and
uncomplicated approach to the condition and
their grandparents.

There is no stigma. No fear. No judgement.

What there IS, is humanity and wisdom beyond their years as we see dementia through the prism of youth.

As Brie says, "Just because you get a diagnosis doesn't mean that you have to stop being the human being that you've always been." Oh Brie, how right you are.

These young people happily inhabit the parallel universe where their grandparents feel safe and in control. They recognise a carer grandmother as being "amazing", intuitively develop "tricks to overcome confusion" and see the end of life approaching like "an old leaf getting ready to fall from the tree".

I think it's brilliant to see Brie, Sam, Fred and Sarah representing a dementia-aware generation who will mature into a society in which dementia is understood, dementia patients are respected and the word "stigma" will no longer be part of the Dementia Dictionary.

These aren't just diaries; they're a real beacon of hope for the future.

— ANGELA

Angela Rippon is Co-Chair Prime Minister's Dementia-Friendly Communities Champion Group, Alzheimer's Society Ambassador

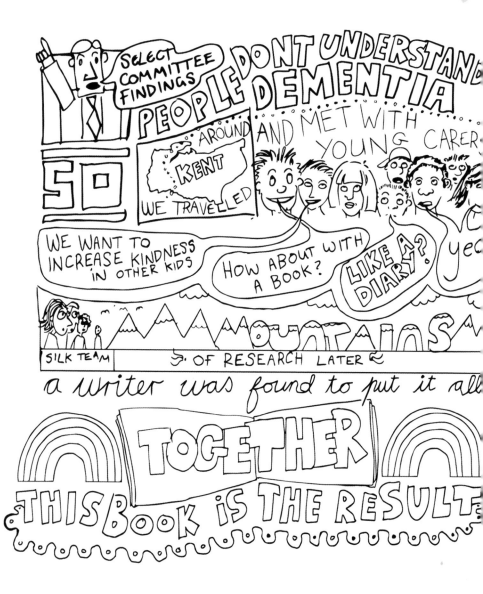

WHERE THIS BOOK HAS BEEN

Thank you for picking this book up. When we started this project, we didn't expect it to be in your hands now.

It all comes from a boy named Jack with a big idea and a huge piece of paper. He was in a session we had with a group of Young Carers in Sittingbourne, Kent. We were tasked with making the region a "Dementia-Friendly Community" as part of the Prime Minister's Challenge. Jack said we needed to make a book about dementia like *Diary of a Wimpy Kid*, or *Adrian Mole*. The group decided we needed to create something for young people "who didn't really know what dementia was", that "did not seem technical and scary" but will give young people an "understanding of dementia and what happens when someone has it". They wanted the journal to be "fiction", but the "**stories should be based on real life**", so that the "**facts are accurate and feelings are real**".

So we worked with families in Kent who were gracious enough to share their stories about living with dementia because they wanted to help others in the future. This book is the result.

And it has taken on a life of its own. We know that this book is already being read and used by healthcare professionals, care providers, teachers and educators, community workers, children and families from London to the Bahamas. The book is currently in every school and library in Kent, Surrey and West Sussex and the Midt Region of Denmark; it is being used with families by Admiral Nurses and dementia charities across the UK and is training social workers and health professionals.

It won an award from the NHS. It was highly commended at the NHS England's Health and Care Expo in 2014, and it has even made it on to the BBC with a special on the *Braincell Boogie*, an animation we produced to accompany the book, which you can find on the Dementia Diaries YouTube channel.

And that's not the end of the story. We've also made a learning resource based on the colourful characters in this book to help bring this book into learning environments. We have included a few activities at the end of each chapter and the rest will be available as a free download via the QR code at the back of this book.

Whatever you use it for, we hope this book supports you to have better relationships with your loved ones. A snippet of information, a story, a smile or a tear, to start a conversation that perhaps otherwise you may not have had.

Please help make a difference – share and connect to our community
@DementiaDiaries
Facebook.com/dementiadiaries

Thank you,
The team and families who created *The Dementia Diaries*

And a special thank you to Jessica Kingsley Publishers, who have taken on the challenge of getting this book into many more hands than we could have ever hoped for.

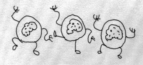

CHAPTER ONE

"I guess sometimes it's just easier to write it down"

Meet Brie, Fred, Sarah and Sam

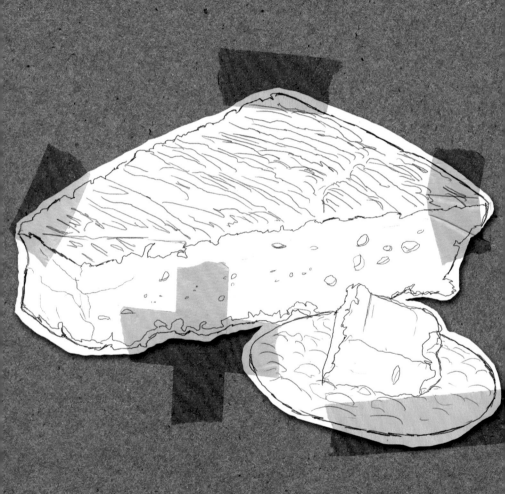

Brie's Diary

Hello. Hi.

My name is Brie. Yes, like the cheese.

I'm 14 years old and I want to share some of my stories with you, the sort of stories that are hard to talk about. But really important. And I want some of my friends to share their stories with you too. Stories about Dementia. Stories about losing someone you love, slowly, one day at a time. Stories about how to remember them as they were, and stories about how to take them as they are.

I don't really know how to just talk about it, and get it out there. I guess sometimes it's just easier to write it down. Make sense of it. To understand what's happening, and maybe even why it's happening.

So yes, that's what this is. It's a diary, it's my diary, and it's my friends' diaries. We've stuck them all together into a sort of super-diary about Dementia.
And it's about our Grandparents.
It's about their Dementia. That's what we want to share.
And don't worry, some of the stories are even pretty funny!

This book is for you, Granddad. And for all the Granddads, and Grannies, and Mums and Dads, and sisters and brothers, and sons and daughters who have met Dementia. You're stronger than you know.

FRED'S NOTEBOOK

RADIO CONTROLLED SUBMARINE

HI, I'M FRED, AND THIS IS MY NOTEBOOK.
I'M NOT CALLING IT A DIARY. IT'S A NOTEBOOK.
DIARIES ARE FOR GIRLS. I THOUGHT I SHOULD START
IT SO I CAN WRITE ABOUT GRAMPS AND HIS DIMENSAS.
WHEN IT'S FULL I'M GONNA BURY IT FOR FUTURE
GENERATIONS. JUST LIKE I DID WITH SIMON'S IPHONE.

PEOPLE SHOULD KNOW ABOUT GRAMPS.
ESPECIALLY FUTURE PEOPLE. LET ME TELL YOU HOW
I FIRST LEARNT ABOUT DIMENSAS. GRAMPS WAS
DRIVING ME AND SIMON TO THE BOATING POND,
SO I COULD TEST OUT THE NEW RADIO
CONTROLLED SUBMARINE HE
GOT ME FOR MY BIRTHDAY.

SUB

SIMON KEPT CHANGING THE CHANNEL ON THE RADIO, HE'S SO ANNOYING. ANYWAY, GRAMPS MADE HIM STOP ON THE NEWS. THEY WERE TALKING ABOUT AN OLD LADY WHO COULDN'T REMEMBER HER CHILDREN, OR EVEN HER GRANDCHILDREN.
CAN YOU IMAGINE THAT? THE WOMAN TALKING ABOUT HER WAS CRYING.
I THINK IT WAS HER DAUGHTER. WHY WOULD THEY PUT THAT ON THE RADIO?

GRAMPS SAW I WEREN'T HAPPY, SO HE SWITCHED IT BACK TO THE CHART SHOW.

WHEN WE GOT THE BOATING LAKE, I'D KIND OF FORGOTTEN ABOUT IT, BECAUSE I WAS SO EXCITED ABOUT MY RADIO CONTROLLED SUBMARINE.
WHICH IS AMAZING. IT'S SO COOL. WE STAYED OUT AT THE POND ATTACKING OTHER KIDS' BOATS UNTIL THEY ALL WENT HOME AND IT GOT COLD.

IT WAS LIKE THE BEST DAY EVER.

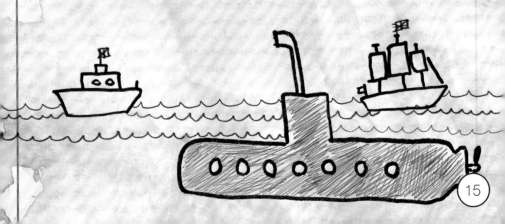

THEN GRAMPS SAID MUM WOULD GET MAD IF WE
WEREN'T BACK FOR DINNER. SO WE WALKED BACK TO
THE CAR AND HE GAVE ME ONE OF THE THREE
JUMPERS THAT HE WEARS.

THAT'S WHEN HE TOLD ME...

HE SAID, "FRED, THAT REPORT ON THE RADIO,
THAT'S WHAT I HAVE. BUT I DON'T WANT YOU TO
WORRY ABOUT ANYTHING. I WILL ALWAYS CONTINUE
TO DO THINGS LIKE THIS WITH YOU FOR AS
LONG AS I POSSIBLY CAN."

I TOLD HIM IT WAS OKAY.

AND THAT HE COULD HAVE
MY SUBMARINE IF HE LIKED...

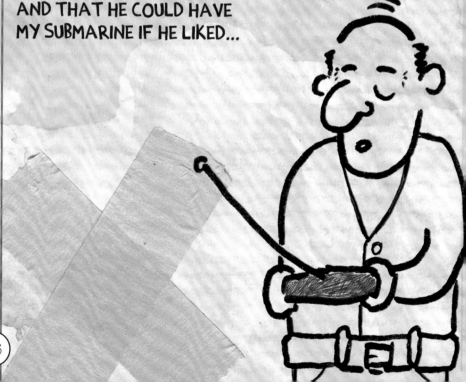

HE JUST PATTED ME ON THE HEAD. THE CAR TRIP HOME WAS REALLY QUIET. SIMON JUST PUT THE MUSIC UP REAL LOUD, AND THEN HE RAN UP TO HIS ROOM AS SOON AS WE GOT HOME.

I'M GLAD GRAMPS TOLD ME. I HOPE HE DOESN'T FORGET US LIKE THE OLD LADY ON THE RADIO. I ASKED MUM SOME MORE ABOUT IT.

SHE SAID IT'S CALLED DEMENSIAS.

I'M GOING TO HAVE TO GOOGLE THAT.

I HOPE HE GETS BETTER SOON, AND THAT HE DOESN'T MOVE VERY VERY FAR AWAY LIKE NANA DID.

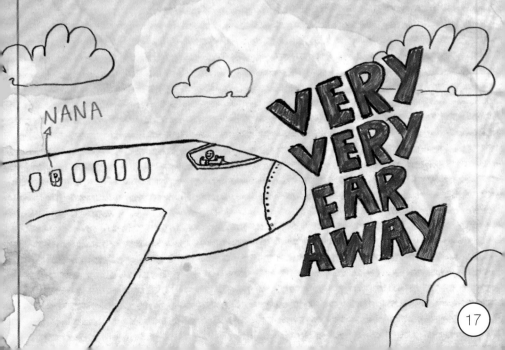

THIS DIARY BELONGS TO

SARAH

LOCAL CELEBRITY

We moved house today. The new house is better, I think. Different. But better.

We're nearer Gran and Grandpa. Well, really near actually. They live across the street!

Mum thinks it's good because Gran and Grandpa are getting well old. I don't know how old exactly. They've been well old as long as I can remember.

Mum wants us to all be here to help. Don't really know what Gran and Grandpa think. But they seem happy to have their granddaughter nearby.

Everyone around here knows Grandpa, he's like a local celebrity or something. They've lived over the road there for 50 years. He used to be a signwriter, and he did all the signs for all them old-fashioned shops in town, so everyone knows him. He even used to do the welcome banners and stagecoaches and that, for when the Royals came to town.

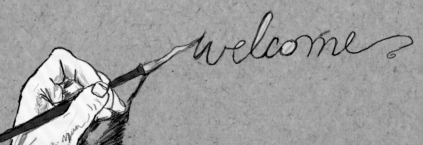

welcome

Everyone knows him and his butcher's bike, rolling down to the High Street to pick up a few bits. I dunno why Mum thinks they need looking after. I think they got more energy than I got! Grandpa even painted the tail bits on planes! And apparently there was one time when there were 50 speed boats all lined up down the road for Grandpa to paint. That's a lot of speed boats.

After we got all our stuff unpacked Grandpa took me for a walk. It was really cool, really interesting. He told me all about all the different places and where he'd lived through the war and stuff. He likes his war stories and history stuff. Last year he was even the special guest at the local Service Club which he founded.

We even went for fish and chips.

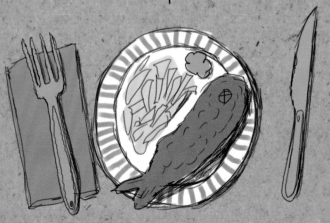

SAM'S DIARY

written by Sam

me

AEROPLANE

MY NAME'S SAM AND I AM 9 AND A HALF YEARS OLD AND I HAVE AN AEROPLANE.

I HAD AN AEROPLANE.

NANNY CRASHED IT ONTO THE ROOF OF THE COMMUNITY CENTRE. WE WAS ALL SCREAMING AT HER TO BRING IT BACK DOWN BECAUSE IT WAS ABOUT FORTY FEET IN THE AIR! YOU'RE NOT SUPPOSED TO FLY IT SO HIGH.

40 FEET

BUT NANNY'S A <u>RISK TAKER</u>.

THAT'S WHY IT'S ON THE ROOF. DAD'S HALF WAY UP A LADDER RIGHT NOW, TRYING TO REACH IT. THAT'S MUCH SAFER THAN WHAT NANNY WAS DOING. SHE WAS TRYING TO CLIMB UP ON THE BINS!

SHE WENT OFF TO GET ME SOME SWEETS TO SAY SORRY, BUT WHEN SHE CAME BACK, THE SWEET PACKET WAS EMPTY. ALL THAT WAS LEFT WAS A STICK-ON TATTOO.

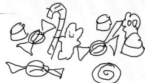

SAM'S DIARY

written by Sam.

AEROPLANE

SHE JUST SAID, "I GOT A SWEET TOOTH." SHE SAYS THAT *EVERY TIME!* IT'S NOT EVEN FUNNY ANYMORE, AND I'M HUNGRY.

sweet tooth.

THIS IS JUST *LIKE* WHEN WE WENT ON HOLIDAY TO THE NEW FOREST AND SHE THREW MY STICKY BALL INTO THE AIR AND IT GOT STUCK ON THE CEILING OF THE CHALET.

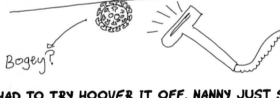

Bogey?

MUM HAD TO TRY HOOVER IT OFF. NANNY JUST SAID MY MASSIVE BOGEY WAS ON THE CEILING.
SHE THINKS SHE'S SO FUNNY, SUCH A BIG JOKER.
IT TOOK TWO DAYS TO FALL OFF THAT CEILING.
TWO DAYS! AND IT LEFT A STAIN.
WASN'T EVEN THAT STICKY AFTERWARDS.

stain

OH THAT'S LUCKY. DAD'S JUST GOT THE PLANE NOW.
I BETTER RUN BEFORE NANNY TRIES TO HAVE ANOTHER GO WITH IT. WHO KNOWS WHERE IT'D END UP.

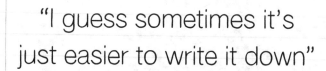

"I guess sometimes it's just easier to write it down"

Chapter One Activities

Memory box

A memory box is a special place to keep important memories. Make a memory box for one of the Dementia Diaries characters or yourself and your family. Include words or objects or pictures from around your house or neighbourhood.

Now, imagine where the characters live. Who lives in a city, who lives near the coast? What are their favourite places to hang out with their friends? Research into what your home town was like 50 years ago and see how it's changed.

Diary

Write a diary entry as yourself or in character, for a favourite memory triggered by the word/object in the memory box.

Radio show

Plan your own radio show! Think about the different types of music people like and create playlists – one for yourself, one for your parents and one for your grandparents.

Share them on Spotify and link to the Dementia Diaries Facebook community (if you already have an account, or ask your parent's permission).

CHAPTER TWO

"Nanny's braincells"

The first signs of dementia

DRIVING LICENCE

Uus Carta de Condução Körkort Riditkļa prkinz Juhilubz Vrdiunje apllotksa Vair Ridiʌkj prūkhʌ Jubitru izymejimen Vexcho eny Vaisuotajo przymejimos Vecobe engeddy Llensgerbz Seudgan Pony. Jazay Vedj Vadcasthy Preukoz Voznisko dovolvenje Adler Odrimarg Perhis de Condicion Cnurenrft. grphuurrn MIICRuuw ao candke Guysoul Cosh uuter mrect

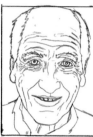

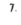

1. c m~~

2. GRANDDAD

3. 09-10-26 ENG
4a. 20-06-12 4b 19-06-22 4c DVLA
5. ~~~610096~ ⅄ ⅄⅃ ~

7. [signature]

8. ~ ~~~

B,BE, C1, C1E, D1, D1E, ſk,ƒ,n,p

BBBBB

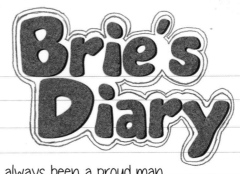

Granddad was a Pharmacist. And he's always been a proud man, so it must have been tough for him to tell us. We were driving somewhere. Well, he was driving. Mary and I were in the back.

We never knew when was the right time to speak with him. When to start the conversation. We were somewhere between Tunstall and Sittingbourne, I think.

Out in the countryside.

That's when we had the accident...

What we found out later was that part of the condition is that you don't always see the thing in front of you, and it affects everybody differently. Granddad turned out into traffic and he didn't see the oncoming car, so it was... it could have been a life-threatening situation.

The other car only hit the bumper a little bit at the front. We were frightened because Granddad just didn't know which way to go or how, or what to do.

We called Grannie. She came to get us.

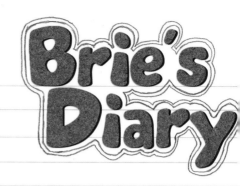

When we got back to theirs, Grannie was saying we need to file the documents to get rid of Granddad's driving licence, and he was a bit angry about that because he knew what was happening, and he was a bit upset that he was losing his driving licence.

I think it was a sensible thing to do. So he could be safer, because he was starting to lose track of sometimes where he was or something. That's why he pulled out in front of that car.

After he had a chat with Grannie, he sat us down in the kitchen, and he couldn't really... He just sort of lost track of what he was saying, and he couldn't get the words out, and then after about 5 minutes of trying he eventually said,

"Oh I can't carry the conversation on. I have Dementia."

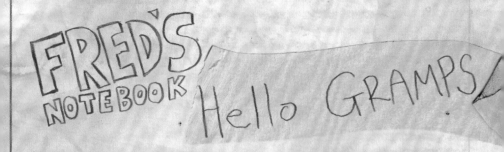

FRED'S NOTEBOOK

Hello GRAMPS!

TODAY GRAMPS MOVED IN WITH US. HE'S NOT HAPPY ABOUT IT. I'M NOT HAPPY ABOUT IT NEITHER. MUM AND DAD MADE ME MOVE INTO SIMON'S ROOM!

NOW GRAMPS IS IN MY ROOM. I HAD TO TAKE DOWN ALL MY POSTERS, AND MOVE ALL MY STUFF.

BUT AT LEAST NOW I'M CLOSER TO SIMON'S X-BOX. ALTHOUGH HE STILL DON'T LIKE ME PLAYING ON IT.

GRAMPS STUFF

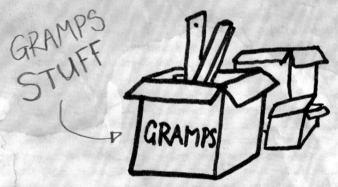

MUM SAYS IT WON'T BE FOR LONG, JUST UNTIL WE FIND A BETTER SITUATION FOR HIM. SHE SAYS HE'S GOT DIMENSAS, AND SINCE NANA MOVED VERY VERY FAR AWAY HE'S BEEN GETTING WORSE. I DID A WIKIPEDIA SEARCH FOR DIMENSIAS.

IT'S ACTUALLY CALLED **DEMENTIA**

TAKE THAT MUM. IT MEANS, "A SERIOUS LOSS OF GLOBAL COGNITIVE ABILITY IN A PREVIOUSLY UNIMPAIRED PERSON, BEYOND WHAT MIGHT BE EXPECTED FROM NORMAL AGEING."

WELL, SOMETIMES HE IS A BIT LOOPY AND A BIT MAD AND HE USUALLY WEARS QUITE A LOT OF CLOTHES, AND HE LIKES WAKING UP A BIT EARLY IN THE MORNING. APART FROM THAT,
I HAVEN'T NOTICED ANY LOSS OF BRAIN STUFF.

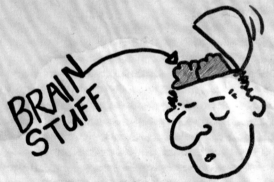

BRAIN STUFF

ANYWAY HE WAS GRUMBLING ALL MORNING. ME AND SIMON EVEN HAD TO CARRY ALL HIS STUFF INTO MY OLD ROOM. HE'S GOT A LOT OF PUZZLES FOR A GROWN-UP. AND CROSSWORD BOOKS. GRAMPS SAYS THEY HELP HIM CONNECT THE DOTS. I DUNNO WHY HE'S TRYING TO CONNECT DOTS IN A CROSSWORD PUZZLE, BUT I GUESS THAT'S JUST GRAMPS.

ANYWAY, HE DIDN'T HAVE THAT MUCH STUFF. I THINK
I HAVE MORE STUFF. I ALWAYS THOUGHT THE OLDER
YOU GOT, THE MORE STUFF YOU'D HAVE. AND WHEN
YOU'RE REALLY OLD YOU'D HAVE LIKE ALL THE STUFF.
GRAMPS SAID ALL THE STUFF WAS IN STORAGE,
AND TO STOP ASKING HIM STUPID QUESTIONS.

AFTER LUNCH HE MADE US WATCH AN OLD WAR
MOVIE. IT HAD LOADS OF SHOOTING.
IT WAS AMAZING.

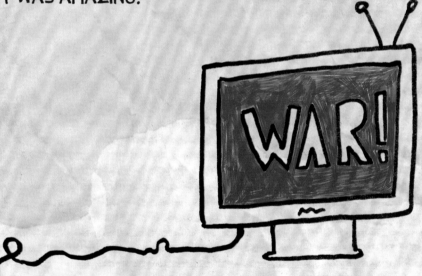

I CAN'T BELIEVE MUM LET US WATCH IT WITH HIM.
IT WAS LIKE CALL OF DUTY ON SIMON'S X-BOX.
BUT LIKE OLD. GRAMPS SAID HE WAS IN THE WORLD
WAR 2, AND THAT THE MOVIE WAS JUST LIKE IT.

I THOUGHT GRAMPS WAS AN INSURANCE SALESMAN,
BUT I GUESS THERE WAS LOTS OF THINGS TO INSURE
IN THE WORLD WAR 2. MUST HAVE BEEN WELL
EXCITING FOR INSURANCE SALESMEN.

ACTUALLY I THINK GRAMPS STAYING WITH US MIGHT
BE NOT SO BAD. EVEN THOUGH HE HAS MY ROOM AND
SIMON SNORES, I THINK HE MIGHT BE A LOT OF FUN.

TODAY GRAMPS CAME TO PICK US UP FROM SCHOOL.
AND WHEN HE STEPPED OUT OF THE CAR, HE WASN'T
WEARING ANY TROUSERS!

SIMON WAS THERE WITH ALL HIS COOL FRIENDS.
IT WAS HILARIOUS. HE WENT BRIGHT RED AND TRIED
TO HIDE.

GRAMPS COULDN'T STOP LAUGHING.
ME NEITHER.

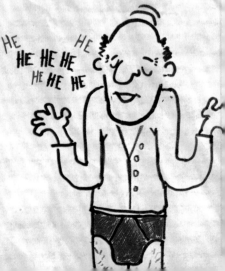
HE HE HE HE HE HE HE

SARAH

THE BAD NEWS

I feel bad, I haven't written in this thing for a while. Not since we moved in, I think, and that was like a year ago. You know when you move house and you put things away, but then you put them away so well that you can't ever find them again? I sort of did that to this diary.

I'm glad I've found it again. There's finally something to write about. Before it was like "Yay, I moved house, how interesting." But now there's something that I feel I really need to put into words.

Grandpa has Alzheimer's.

We found out a few months ago. It was quite slow at first, he's only 77 years old. I thought you only got Alzheimer's when you were like 90 years old.

I used to think you spelt Alzheimer's, "Oldtimers." That made sense to me.

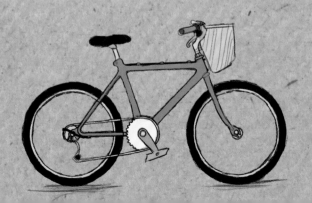

THIS DIARY BELONGS TO
SARAH

We had to stop him from riding his bike down to the High Street. Because it was such an old bike, we told him that we can't get the parts for it anymore!

Luckily he believed us. He was such a danger to himself and other people and traffic. Because you've got the main road right there, there'd be traffic going past, and Grandpa thought you could just pull out into the road without looking or stopping.

He still does his walks though. Because of the Alzheimer's, he goes down the town every day and he always buys a loaf of bread, a carrot and a potato.

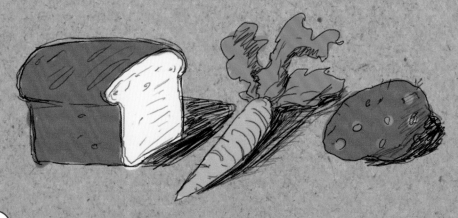

THIS DIARY BELONGS TO
SARAH

It's such a regular thing now that if he hadn't been down the town for his carrot; the shops would be ringing up asking, "is your Grandpa alright, he's not been in for his carrot today?"

It's really good that's he's such a local celebrity, because even all the kids know Grandpa.

Like I'll get a text, or someone would knock on the door, and they'd say that they'd seen him out down the park, or he's down the seafront. Everyone knows that he likes to wander and everyone keeps an eye out, which is really nice.

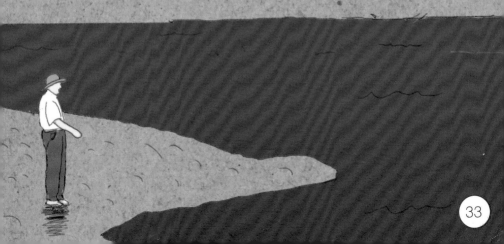

SAM'S DIARY

written by Sam

NANNY'S BRAIN CELLS

SOMEONE ASKED ME IF NANNY'S CHANGED IN THE LAST
FEW YEARS. I DON'T KNOW, I'M ONLY NINE.
I CAN'T REMEMBER THAT FAR BACK.
BUT I THINK NANNY IS AS SILLY AS EVER.
SHE SAYS IT'S BECAUSE SHE'S SO
OLD SHE'S ONLY GOT TWO BRAIN CELLS LEFT.

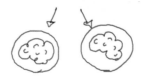

AND MUM SAID THAT WHEN YOU SNEEZE YOU LOSE ONE
BRAIN CELL, SO NANNY'S GOT MINUS BRAINCELLS NOW!!
BUT YEAH I KNOW SHE'S GETTING OLD AND
THAT, BUT I DON'T SEE IT.

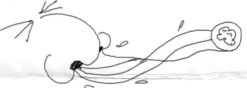

I LOOK AT MY SCHOOL PHOTO FROM YEAR THREE AND
I LOOK WELL YOUNG, BUT NANNY PROBABLY LOOKED
THE SAME THEN AS SHE DOES NOW. I THINK YOU'RE
OLD FROM WHEN YOU'RE LIKE 30, THEN YOU JUST GET
MORE WRINKLES. AND SOMETIMES YOU FORGET THAT
YOU'RE OLD. I THINK NANNY'S FORGOT THAT SHE'S OLD.

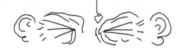

SAM'S DIARY
written by SAM

NANNY'S BRAIN CELLS

THAT'S WHY SHE KEEPS EATING MY SWEETS AND
NICKING MY TOYS. I TRIED TO TRICK HER INTO
GIVING ME SOME EXTRA POCKET MONEY THE
OTHER DAY.

I TOLD HER SHE PROMISED. BUT SHE KNEW.
INSTEAD SHE GAVE ME ANOTHER EMPTY PACKET OF
SWEETS AND A STICK-ON TATTOO, AND SHE SAID,
"YOU'RE GOING TO GET ME ONE DAY, BUT THAT
DAY IS NOT TODAY." I THINK I SHOULD KEEP TRYING.

IT WAS WEIRD THE OTHER DAY WHEN WE WENT TO
THIS CAMPSITE FOR EASTER. NANNY AND ME WENT
FOR A WALK, WHILE MUM AND DAD AND THEM LOT
WAS COOKING DINNER.

SAM'S DIARY
written by Sam

NANNY'S BRAIN CELLS

AND THEN WE WENT A LITTLE WAYS THROUGH THE
WOODS AND WAS LOOKING AT SOME FROGS, AND THEN
NANNY BUMPED INTO SOME PEOPLE SHE KNEW AND IT
WAS BLAH BLAH BLAH...

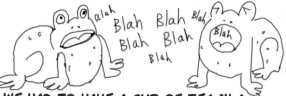

THEN WE HAD TO HAVE A CUP OF TEA IN A
CARAVAN SOMEWHERE. IT WAS WELL BORING.
ANYWAY IT WAS GETTING DARK AND WE HEARD
PEOPLE CALLING OUR NAMES. THEY'D ONLY
GONE AND MADE A SEARCH PARTY! THEY SAID THEY
WERE LOOKING FOR US EVERYWHERE. IT'S JUST DINNER,
WHAT'S SO IMPORTANT ABOUT DINNER THAT THEY
HAVE TO SEND OUT A SEARCH PARTY!

I KNOW MUM THINKS SHE'S A GOOD COOK, BUT
SHE'S NOT THAT GOOD! NANNY SAID THEY WERE ALL
PANICKY FOR NOTHING. BUT IT DID GET ME OUT OF
HAVING TEA WITH THOSE OLD WRINKLY PEOPLE.
NANNY SAYS NEXT TIME WE'LL DO A PROPER
ADVENTURE WALK, HOPEFULLY WITH MORE FROGS.

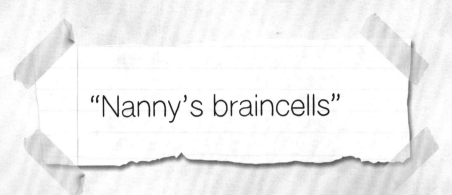

"Nanny's braincells"

Chapter Two Activities

Email

Imagine you are one of the characters. How would you write an email to a friend or a member of your family to tell them The News. Remember to include the name of their grandparent, how they found out, the symptoms that their grandparent has, how they react to the news and how they feel.

Poster

Make a poster about dementia. Think about who the audience will be. Is it for a public place or a school, hospital, library or somewhere else? Include information about dementia and the different forms it can take.

ID Card

Design a form of ID for a person living with dementia who may be prone to getting lost or going missing. What is the important information that it needs to have on it?

Map

Imagine you are Sarah. Draw a map to show the route Grandpa usually walks every day.

Storyboard

Draw a storyboard for the incident with Sam and his Nanny. Either recreate the storyboard from his point of view or from the point of view one of the people they met on their walk.

Talk

Discuss how Gramps' behaviour is changing. What are Fred's family doing to support him?

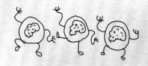

CHAPTER THREE

"Puzzled"

Ways of coping with dementia

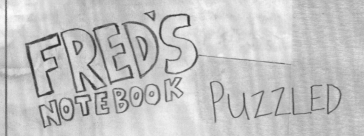

PUZZLED

GRAMPS IS SO FUNNY ABOUT HIS TIME. HE WILL ONLY EAT BREAKFAST IF IT'S 8.30 IN THE MORNING.

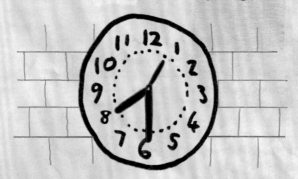

OTHERWISE HE WON'T TOUCH IT. MUM TRIED TO CHANGE THE CLOCKS ON THE WALL TO TRICK HIM, BUT HE STILL HAD HIS WRISTWATCH ON.
I GUESS IT'S GOOD THAT WE CAN'T TRICK HIM LIKE THAT YET.

I THINK IT'S REALLY CLEVER. I'M GOING TO DO IT TO SIMON'S NEW PHONE.

GRAMPS LIKES TO STICK TO HIS SCHEDULE.
IT'S VERY IMPORTANT TO HIM.

HE DOESN'T REALLY LIKE EATING WITH US, BECAUSE WE'RE NOT ALWAYS THERE ON TIME. HE GETS LESS STRESSED IF IT'S JUST HIM EATING.

MUM SAYS IF HE DOESN'T EAT AT HIS TIMES, IT THROWS HIM FOR THE WHOLE DAY, SO WE TRY TO KEEP TO HIS ROUTINE. SOMETIMES FOR SPECIAL OCCASIONS I GUESS WE DO EAT WITH HIM.

BUT WE HAVE TO BE THERE SITTING DOWN AT THE RIGHT TIME. FOR LUNCH IT'S 12 O'CLOCK AND DINNER IS AT 6.30PM. BUT WEIRDLY, ON SUNDAYS HE DOESN'T MIND WHEN HE EATS, BECAUSE IT'S A SUNDAY, I GUESS.

ALSO HE GOES TO HIS CLUB ON TUESDAYS AND SUNDAYS. AFTER BREAKFAST HE NORMALLY GOES TO THE LIVING ROOM AND WORKS ON HIS CROSSWORDS. HE REALLY DOES THEM EVERY DAY. SOMETIMES HE GETS US TO HELP. I GET BORED, THERE'S ONLY SO MANY CROSSWORDS YOU CAN DO IN A DAY, SURELY?

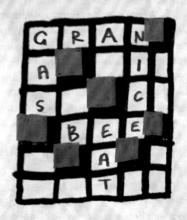

BUT HE ALWAYS MAKES SURE TO FINISH THE ONES HE STARTS. SOME OF THEM HAVE BEEN SITTING OUT FOR LIKE A WEEK. I THINK HE MAKES IT HARD FOR HIMSELF BY USING A PEN. CAN'T CHEAT WITH A PEN! NORMALLY WE JUST STICK ON A MOVIE OR A CARTOON.

SIMON JUST GOES UPSTAIRS TO TALK TO HIS GIRLFRIEND ON THE PHONE. I DON'T KNOW IF I WANT TO BE A TEENAGER. GIRLS SEEM LIKE QUITE A LOT OF HARD WORK.

AFTER LUNCH IS USUALLY GRAMPS' PUZZLE TIME. HE'S BEEN WORKING ON THIS ONE PUZZLE OF THE ROYAL FAMILY FOR AGES AND HE CAN'T SEEM TO FIND THE RIGHT PIECES. THE OTHER DAY HE CAME INTO THE KITCHEN AND SHOWED US A PUZZLE PIECE AND SAID, "IT'S A DOG" WHEN IT WAS THE QUEEN WITH HER GLASSES ON.

IT WAS SO FUNNY.

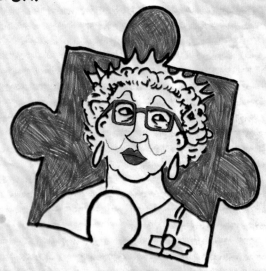

MUM SAYS HE KEEPS DOING THESE PUZZLES
AND CROSSWORDS TO KEEP HIS BRAIN MOVING,

TO FIGHT OFF THE DEMENTIA.

I THINK IT'S GOOD HE WANTS TO FIGHT IT. IT MUST
BE REALLY SCARY TO KEEP FORGETTING THINGS,
AND HAVING YOUR MIND IN A BIG JUMBLE.

I THINK IT'S A BIT LIKE HIS PUZZLES;

BECAUSE HE KEEPS LOSING PIECES, AND EVERY DAY
IT'S LIKE HE'S TRYING TO PUT HIMSELF BACK
TOGETHER AGAIN.

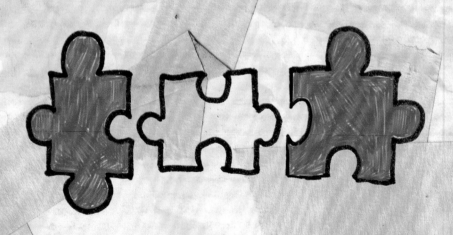

THIS DIARY BELONGS TO
SARAH
MISSING PERSON

Grandpa disappeared at 4 o'clock yesterday. He was in one of his bad moods and nobody could talk him out of it. He sometimes has his little outbursts.
It depends on the weather and things like that, I think. But anyway, he just went to the bathroom and climbed out the window, and then he went off trotting down the road. They say when someone with Alzheimer's is on a mission they're just off on one. He could shuffle pretty far if he wanted to.

And it was getting dark.

Me and Mum went down to town and we were going to all the stores saying, "Grandpa's gone walkabout and we don't know where he is." Luckily, because he's such a local celebrity, we didn't have to stand around and do descriptions because everyone knows what he looks like. And everyone was looking for him!

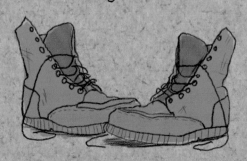

There was like 4 police cars and 3 or 4 PCSOs, and about 10 people from the police and what have you, and like 8 family members. I guess because we're so close to the coast and surrounded by fields, everyone was worried about the cold. It was freezing out. The police were on about getting Search and Rescue in. We were all so worried about him. Gran especially.

We thought maybe we should check the house one more time before we called the Search and Rescue lads in, so we headed to Gran and Grandpa's house... and you know what? There he was! He'd managed to sneak back home without anyone noticing. One of the neighbours had been watching the house as a lookout! And Grandpa was fast asleep in his chair! It was such a relief.

When we found him there, one of my aunties started yelling at him, saying that he'd done wrong and telling him off. I think she was just scared and a little bit angry. But you can't tell them off, you can't shout or raise your voice, you've just got to relax and accept them as they are.

SARAH

Fast forward to this morning, and Mum and Gran came up with a plan. They've installed cameras in the house, so we can check on him from ours on the computer. Like if he needs help or he's wandered off or anything. They've even got a tracker in his trousers so they can see where he is. I think the tracker's a really good idea, especially because this morning he disappeared again...

He wandered off and he wasn't on the park bench like he normally was, so me and Bob (my dog) was out walking looking for him, and he'd set the tracker off and so we knew whereabouts to go. He was walking towards the coast and we found him on Sea Road, by the beach, sat on a bench. When we got there he looked at us and went, "Hello, what are you doing 'ere?"

So he doesn't find out about the tracker I told him this was where we were planning to meet all along.
He seemed to believe it luckily.
I don't like lying to him, but I guess it's for his own good. I called Mum to pick us up and take Grandpa home.

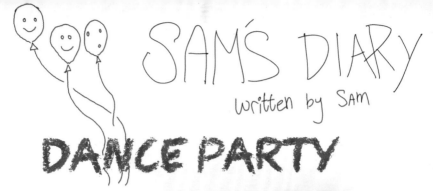

SAM'S DIARY

written by Sam

DANCE PARTY

FOR NANNY'S BIRTHDAY THIS YEAR WE ALL WENT ON A
HOLIDAY TO THE NEW FOREST AGAIN. NANNY LOVES IT
THERE. IT WAS ME, MUM, DAD AND GRANDAD AND NANNY.
EVERY NIGHT WE WERE THERE, NANNY WANTED TO GO
DANCING. SHE WANTED TO DANCE IN THE RESTAURANT, IN
THE PUB, IN THE WOODS.
EVERYWHERE!

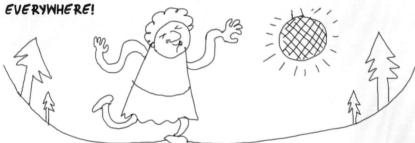

SO EVERYONE WENT DANCING LIKE EVERY NIGHT.
AND THEY KEPT ON DANCING AT THIS DISCO THING.
I JOINED IN THE SONGS SOMETIMES BUT MOST OF THE
TIME I PLAYED ON MUM'S SAMSUNG GALAXY.
FOR OLD PEOPLE, THEY SURE LIKE TO BOOGIE.
I LIKE DANCING TO MICHAEL JACKSON.
I'M TRYING TO LEARN HOW TO MOONWALK,
I'VE BEEN WATCHING IT ON YOUTUBE,
BUT I HAVEN'T FIGURED IT OUT YET.
NANNY CAN DO IT. SHE'S GOT SKILLS,
THE REST OF THEM ARE A
BIT RUBBISH.

SAM'S DIARY

written by SAM

DANCE PARTY

ANYWAY I THINK THEY MUST HAVE DANCED ALL NIGHT. I
HAD A NAP FOR A BIT, AND WHEN I WOKE UP THEY WERE
STILL DANCING.

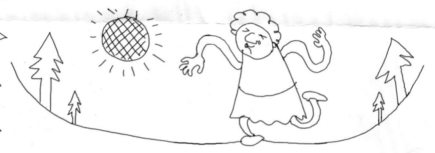

WE'RE JUST A DANCING FAMILY, I GUESS. THEY HAD
THESE OLD BOTTLES OF RIBENA THAT THEY KEPT TO
THEMSELVES. I DON'T KNOW WHY THEY WOULDN'T LET ME
HAVE ANY. GRANDAD SAID IT WASN'T FOR LITTLE KIDS
AND WOULD PROBABLY PUT HAIR ON MY CHEST.

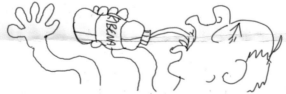

RIBENA? I DRINK RIBENA LIKE EVERY DAY, AND I STILL
DON'T GET ANY HAIR ON MY CHEST!

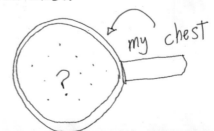

my chest

?

SAM'S DIARY
written by Sam

DANCE PARTY

I LOVE MY FAMILY. THERE WAS SOME FAMILIES THERE
THAT DIDN'T DANCE AT ALL. LIKE THEY WERE SCARED OF
DANCING OR SOMETHING?! WE DON'T CARE.

WE JUST DANCE, AND WHEN THEM LOT ALL LEAVE AND
THERE'S NOBODY LEFT ON THE DANCE FLOOR, NANNY
SAYS THAT'S THE BEST TIME TO SMASH IT. AND THEN
SHE BOOGIES AND DOES HER MOONWALKS AND STUFF.
MY FAMILY LIKES TO SING TOO. NOT WELL.

LA LA LA LA LA LA LA LA

BUT IF EVERYONE'S DOING IT, YOU DON'T WANT TO BE A
BILLY-NO-MATES, ESPECIALLY ON A HOLIDAY.
SO WE WERE ALL SINGING AND DANCING TO MICHAEL
JACKSON ON NANNY'S BIRTHDAY. IT WAS <u>WICKED</u>.!!

THE NEXT MORNING EVERYONE WAS KNACKERED. NANNY
SAID SHE WAS "YOUNG AT HEART" BUT THAT SHE
NEEDED A HOLIDAY TO GET OVER THE HOLIDAY, MUM
JUST GROANED AND PUT HER SUNGLASSES ON.

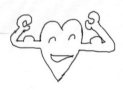

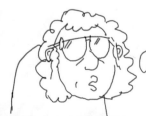

GROOOaaahn

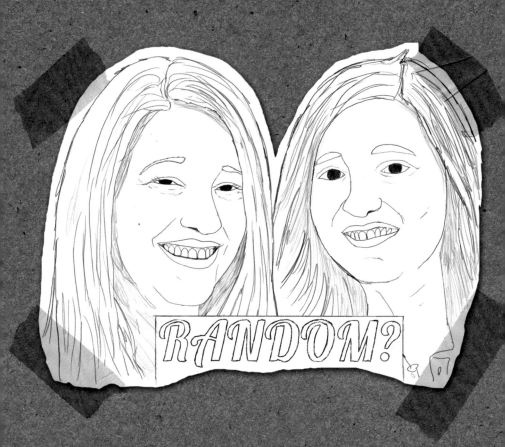

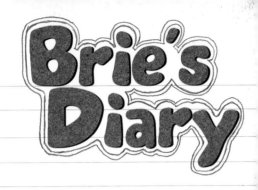

Brie's Diary

I'm at Grannie and Granddad's flat in Eastborne again this weekend...
I can literally see the seaside through the window as I write this.
It's so random. I used to love coming down here, but that was back
when the Dementia was first starting. I actually don't remember that
part very well, but I do remember Granddad was a bit forgetting what
he was doing. I suppose that probably only started a bit later but
I don't remember the really really beginning, you know.

I remember he would sometimes take us to our favourite cafe, by the
little green before the cliff. I used to be a little bit scared of him,
we all were. Well, scared isn't the right word. We were intimidated.
He was always so smart, and intellectual-like.

When me and my sisters would sit with him and Grannie at the cafe,
it would always get really quiet. Granddad would always be reading his
newspaper, in a very serious way.

I don't think anyone could read a newspaper as seriously as Granddad
could. And Grannie would have a book. I don't think they were used
to three little 7- and 8-year-old girls. We were always sitting opposite
each other trying not to laugh at how serious Granddad looked, and
that just got us into hysterics all the time. It would get him really
annoyed.

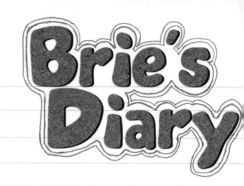

But I think maybe it was quiet because he was probably waiting for the time when we were old enough to understand half of the things he was trying to talk to us about, and have a more intellectual conversation than our 8-year-old knowledge.

Sometimes he would try. He'd talk about things like Science and gravity. Very clever conversations about certain topics.

I remember one trip down here we were trying to get someone to give us the definition of the word random. Because we could never find anybody to give us the definition. When we asked Granddad, he literally gave us an answer just that like that, and he said "irregular" which I've always remembered, it's one thing I'll always remember.

And then we were so surprised we didn't really have anything to say after that. We'd been looking for an answer and we thought we were really really clever having this one word which no-one could define, and then he did straight away. He was so clever.

Anyway, what was I going to write about again?
Oh yes.
Today was a good day...

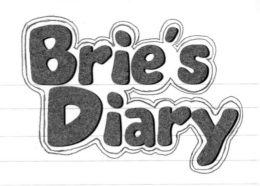

We thought we'd go for a walk like in the old days, down to the cafe and the fish and chip shop by the little green before the cliff. Even walking's a bit of a worry there because it's so easy to trip over the bumpy pavements.

Well, when we got to the cafe, there were some boys playing football on the green and the football came towards us and Granddad ran over to kick it, and I was really really worried that he was going to miss it or fall over or something, it was really worrying. He got it which was nice but it was quite worrying. I don't think he'd like me worrying! He'd probably tell me off.

I think it's quite difficult because now he can't talk and he can't really move much or do anything I suppose, unfortunately, so Grannie says talk to him like you would anyone else as if he was there in the room and always make sure you include him.

It's hard because I don't think I ever got to have any real good conversations with him. Mary did, but she's older. She was always good at having conversations with him. So I thought I would try to talk about intellectual things, but like easy things. Like what I want to do when I'm older, that sort of stuff.

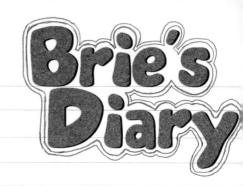

He wouldn't like you just wittering on randomly and now I'm quite conscious when I'm talking to him that I must just witter on about random things. In fact I say I'm really sorry if I'm wittering on about my random life because I know he won't appreciate that, but I also don't want to sound like i'm being patronising.

But when I said that, my random life, he smiled. Like he remembered telling me the definition.

It was easier then. I know everyone's different but if you don't really know how to act or what to do around someone like my Granddad, I think it's good to be the same as usual.

Because deep down, they are too.

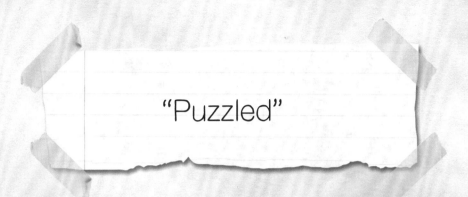

"Puzzled"

Chapter Three Activities

Make a game

How is Gramps trying to keep his mind active? How do you keep your mind active? Create your own crossword, wordsearch or snap cards, or make up your own puzzle. Write a simple list of instructions.

Search and rescue

Make a "missing poster" for Grandpa that could be used by a search and rescue team. Think about the pros and cons of the assistive technology – cameras and a tracker – used to support Grandpa. How do you think Grandpa would be feeling?

Feelings

How do you think people living with dementia feel?
Think about their emotions and why they might feel this way?

Braincell Boogie

Watch the Braincell Boogie on YouTube.
What is the advice about supporting people living with dementia?

Write your own Braincell Boogie poem, song or rhyme. Share your new version on the Dementia Diaries Facebook community pages.

Act

Write your own short play about a person living with dementia.
How would you set the scene?

CHAPTER FOUR

"Shirt, jumper, shirt, jumper, shirt, jumper, cardigan"

Things change as dementia progresses

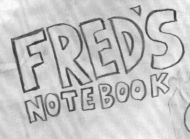

FRED'S NOTEBOOK

GRAMPS' CLUB

THE FIRST RULE OF GRAMPS' CLUB IS NO KIDS.

SO ME AND SIMON HAVE NEVER BEEN. GRAMPS LOVES IT THOUGH. I BET THEY DO A LOT OF CROSSWORDS AND WATCH WAR MOVIES ALL THE TIME!

I CAN'T EVEN IMAGINE HOW MANY CROSSWORD BOOKS THEY MUST HAVE.

GRAMPS IS ALWAYS SMILING WHEN HE COMES BACK, EXCEPT FOR WHEN THE FOOD'S NOT SO GOOD. BUT THEY'VE GOT BETTER, HE SAYS. MUM GAVE THEM A LIST OF THE FOOD HE LIKES. CLEVER MUM!

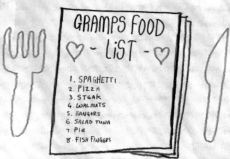

GRAMPS FOOD
♡ - LIST - ♡

1. SPAGHETTI
2. PIZZA
3. STEAK
4. WALNUTS
5. BANGERS
6. SALAD TUNA
7. PIE
8. FISH FINGERS

I WONDER IF EVERYONE AT THE CLUB HAS TO SIT DOWN FOR LUNCH AT 12 O'CLOCK WITH HIM TOO. I THINK PROBABLY.

THEY SURPRISED HIM ON TUESDAY WHEN THEY CAME TO FETCH HIM. HE THOUGHT IT WAS MONDAY. HE WASN'T READY YET. THEY HAD TO WAIT FOR HIM IN THE BUS. THIS IS STARTING TO HAPPEN MORE AND MORE, HIM MISSING THINGS, OR LOSING TRACK OF TIME. HE'S GOT SOME MEDICINE NOW,

WHICH IS HELPING HIM, I THINK. THE TRICK WHERE WE CHANGE THE CLOCK ON THE WALL TO HIS BREAKFAST TIME REALLY WORKS NOW. I DON'T KNOW IF THAT MAKES ME HAPPY OR SAD. HE'S ALSO STARTED CALLING ME SIMON NOW, WHICH IS THE WORST THING.

MUM SAID THEY GOT HIM DANCING AT THE CLUB LAST WEEK. GRAMPS DANCING! NO WAY. HE'S NOT A DANCER. HE'S AN INSURANCE SALESMAN. INSURANCE SALESMEN DON'T DANCE, DO THEY? DEFINITELY NOT GRAMPS. THAT MUST HAVE BEEN HILARIOUS. HE WAS TELLING EVERYONE HE'S FROM BRAZIL! BUT HE'S FROM TUNBRIDGE WELLS! UNLESS THERE'S A TUNBRIDGE WELLS IN BRAZIL THAT I DON'T KNOW ABOUT, BUT I DON'T THINK THERE IS.

I DON'T THINK MANY BRAZILIANS WEAR THREE SHIRTS, THREE JUMPERS, AND A CARDIGAN EITHER.

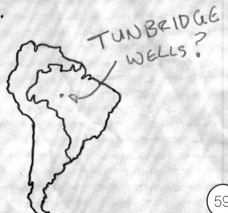

TUNBRIDGE WELLS?

THIS DIARY BELONGS TO
SARAH
SCARECROWS

So after Grandpa's last little adventure with the police search team and all (and the fact that he can't find his way home even in his own road, which has only got thirty houses and he's lived there for over fifty years!), Mum thought it'd be good if I took Grandpa for more walks. It sort of ended up being a role reversal. Grandpa used to take me for walks and now I take my Grandpa for walks!

It's got to the stage where he keeps getting lost so often that it's good to have someone walk with him. Although he still thinks he's taking me for the walks! We take Bobby too, because he loves being off the lead, down the green, chasing his ball.

Grandpa likes to sit on the bench and watch me throw the ball for Bobby. He's always forgetting Bobby's name now. He just calls him Doggy. Close enough, I guess.

After the park we normally walk down to the fish and chip shop. Grandpa likes to keep a pocket full of pennies and things. I always take some money with me but he always insists on paying.

So he gives me the pennies, and insists they're pounds. Pockets full of pounds, he says. I've made a deal with the lads there – we pay in pennies and then on the way out, I sneak back and pay with proper money.

It's tough sometimes when someone greets him, they go, "Oh no, he knows who I am." But he wouldn't know who they was, and it's tough because people believe he's the same as before. But really he can't remember who his own family is. On the way back from the High Street, after we'd got his loaf of bread, carrot and potato, he's always going about seeing the Boss.

"I'm going to see the Boss, I've got to see that man." And you gotta say, "Sorry Grandpa, he's just clocked off. He's just gone home for the night. Let's come back another day." That normally works and then Grandpa's quite happy to head home.

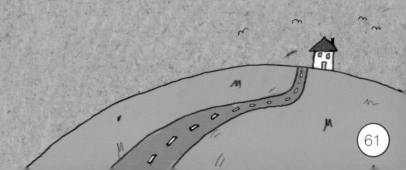

Then there's the scarecrow up at Wyevales.
This life-sized 6 foot scarecrow. Grandpa's got a bit of a beef with this scarecrow. It was fun at the beginning. He used to go in and say hello to it and we'd go along with it and say hello too. Then last week, Grandpa got right in its face and started swearing at it and got really aggressive. He swore a little bit and said the scarecrow hadn't spoke to him again.

Ever since then, I try to take Grandpa on a different route home.
Because every time he sees the scarecrow he puts two fingers right up in its face.

Mum says we should see what he can cope with. Then when he can't cope with something, then we know maybe that we've gone a bit too far. But that don't stop us dragging him around really, shopping, concerts, wherever we need to go.

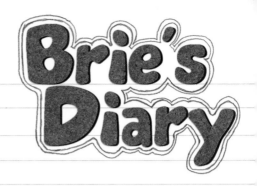

I'm writing from Grannie and Granddad's again today.

It's been really tough on her, so it's good that I'm here, I think.
Another pair of eyes. But it still takes a bit of getting used to.
I don't know, Grannie left me for the afternoon, she went to get her
hair done or something. She's been gone about an hour. Granddad's
been watching the Wimbledon all day. He must have watched all the
matches by now. He really used to like that Andy Murray.

You know, the one who always tries really hard then almost wins.

I can't even be bothered to watch Wimbledon normally, just lots of
people running back and forth and then changing sides. It makes my
head dizzy! Who knows what Granddad must have been thinking.

So I thought, you know maybe I should make an effort, so I started
chatting with him about random stuff. I know I said I mustn't chat
about random stuff with him, only serious stuff. But I was tired and
I couldn't really think of anything good. So I thought I'd tell him about
how Andy Murray won a gold medal at the Olympics, and how the
whole country was smiling for weeks.

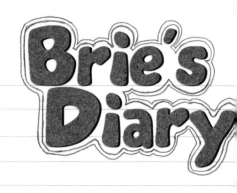

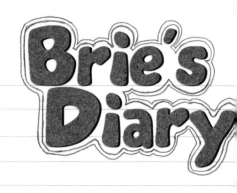

I've sort of gotten used to talking to him like this. It's a bit like talking to someone when they're looking the opposite way… but it's not their fault. To be honest, I find it very difficult to talk to Granddad now because it's just like talking to someone who's not there, unfortunately.

I think that's probably why a lot of his mates don't visit so much anymore. It makes Grannie quite sad. They said they "want to remember him the way he was".

Now, that's really not right because Granddad is still Granddad. He's alive now, and Grannie's alone with him most of, well, all of the time, so where's the support for them both as a couple?! I think people need to get over that. It's like cancer. You don't stop visiting someone because they've got cancer! If anything, you feel, "Oh, well I must keep visiting them even though all their hair has dropped out." You still feel! Granddad's friends have got to get over that fear barrier with Dementia because it can manifest itself so strangely and differently. Maybe that's why they are so frightened of it or whatever.

But just because you get a diagnosis doesn't mean that you have to stop being the human being that you've always been!

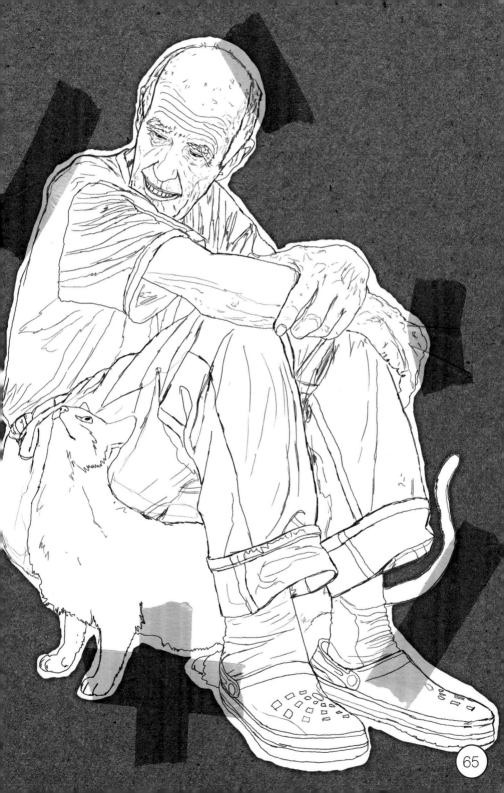

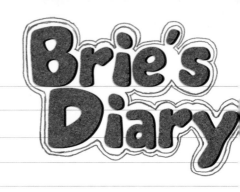

Anyway, Andy Murray. The Olympics.

I tried that for a bit and then I went over to him in his big chair and I switched the TV to mute when the adverts came on, because he used to hate the adverts. Time wasters he called them. And that's when I realised he wasn't watching the TV at all. I don't think he was even listening to me talk about Andy Murray.
There was a cat on the window sill, looking in.

Granddad was watching the cat!

I thought that was a bit random. Granddad's not the sort of person who would ever really have paid much attention to small animals and things, but he was absolutely fascinated.
So I went over to the window and let the cat in.
You should have seen Granddad's face light up!

I've never seen such a big grin! In like two seconds he was trailing a piece of wool along the carpet for the cat. It was just like this childlike pleasure playing with this cat. It was so sweet really. So not like him though. I could never ever imagine Granddad doing this two years ago. I wish he could have seen himself! He would have been shocked!

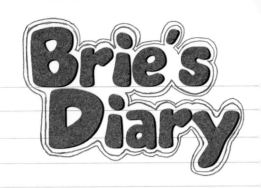

When Grannie got home I told her all about the cat. She said that the cat's been visiting for a few weeks now, and every time it comes over, Granddad plays with it. The cat must be lonely at home, so he comes and visits Granddad for some company. And when Granddad sees the cat, it's like the first time he's ever seen it!

That's a special sort of joy, I think. I think I can understand why that cat keeps coming back. Especially if Granddad does that big grin every time.

I've decided I'm going to remember that grin — that's a grin I'm keeping for myself. I think those sorts of memories are special — even in the sort of darkness of the disease, you can still have these moments of total joy.

And I think that's better than watching Wimbledon any day of the week.

PS. I think I'm going to name the cat Murray.

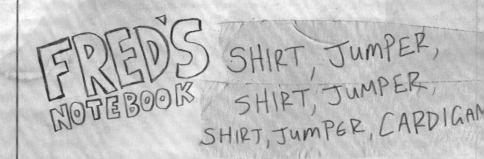

FRED'S NOTEBOOK

SHIRT, JUMPER,
SHIRT, JUMPER,
SHIRT, JUMPER, CARDIGAN

OH BOY. HE'S AT IT AGAIN. IT'S 3 IN THE MORNING. HE'S DOING THE THING AGAIN. HE'S DONE THIS MAYBE TWICE A WEEK SINCE HE MOVED IN WITH US. AND IT'S ALWAYS THE SAME.

YOU CAN TELL IT'S HAPPENING FROM BED 'CAUSE YOU CAN HEAR THE TAP RUNNING IN THE BATHROOM. GRAMPS IS UP, AND HE'S HAVING A SHAVE. THEN HE'S GOING TO GO BACK TO HIS ROOM AND GET DRESSED.

HE'LL PUT ON HIS TROUSERS,
THEN ANOTHER PAIR OF TROUSERS,
AND THEN HE'S GOING TO PUT ON HIS VEST,
THEN A SHIRT,
THEN A JUMPER,
THEN ANOTHER SHIRT,
THEN ANOTHER JUMPER,
THEN ANOTHER SHIRT,
THEN ANOTHER JUMPER,

THEN HIS CARDIGAN!

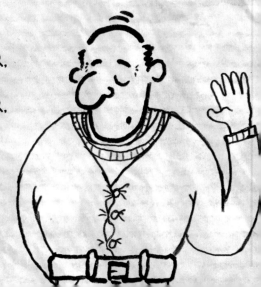

THAT BIT'S ALWAYS THE SAME. SHIRT, JUMPER,
SHIRT, JUMPER, SHIRT, JUMPER, CARDIGAN.

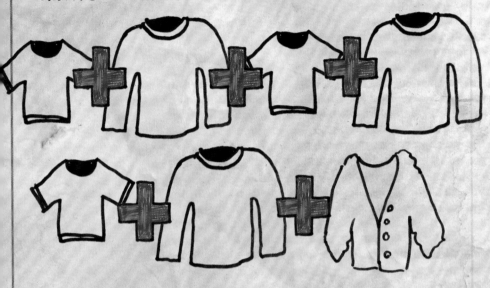

I TRIED IT ONCE, MUM WENT MENTAL. REALLY WARM
THOUGH. THEN TO FINISH IT ALL OFF, HE'S GOING TO
TUCK THE CARDIGAN INTO HIS TROUSERS.

AND HE ALWAYS GETS THE BUTTONS IN THE WRONG
HOLES ON THE CARDIGAN. I DO THAT TOO
SOMETIMES. NOT AS MUCH AS GRAMPS THOUGH.
MUM ALWAYS HAS TO FIX HIS BUTTONS.
IT'S WELL FUNNY.

THEN THE BEST BIT, HE PUTS ON HIS SHOES. AND THEN
HE PUTS ON HIS SOCKS OVER THE SHOES!

I CAN'T EVEN DO THAT. IT'S PROPER AMAZING. MUM
KEEPS HAVING TO BUY HIM NEW SOCKS,

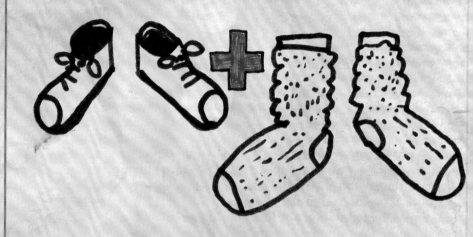

BECAUSE THEY GET SO DIRTY. ESPECIALLY WHEN
HE GOES IN THE GARDEN. THEN AFTER HE PUTS HIS
SHOES AND SOCKS ON, HE'LL GO DOWNSTAIRS AND
HAVE BREAKFAST.

OH THERE IT IS NOW, I CAN HEAR HIM POURING THE
CEREAL. MUM'S PROBABLY AWAKE NOW TOO.

SHE'S GOING TO GET READY AND GO DOWNSTAIRS.
GRAMPS WILL SAY GOOD MORNING, AND THAT HE'S
READY TO GO THE CLUB. MUM WILL FIX HIS BUTTONS
AND THEY'LL GET IN THE CAR. THEN SHE'LL DRIVE
HIM ROUND THE BLOCK AND COME BACK, AND THEN
GRAMPS WILL GO BACK TO BED.

MUM HAS SAID SOMETHING TO HIM ABOUT IT A
COUPLE OF TIMES, BUT HE STILL DOES IT. HE GETS A
BIT STRESSED IF THEY DON'T GO STRAIGHT AWAY.
ONE TIME HE DECIDED TO WALK. AND HE GOT LOST
AND WE COULDN'T FIND HIM. DAD FOUND HIM SITTING
ON THE BENCH IN THE PARK. HE THOUGHT IT WAS THE
BUS STOP! JUST IN CASE IT HAPPENED AGAIN, DAD
PUT A BENCH IN FRONT OF THE HOUSE,
WITH A FAKE BUS STOP SIGN.

ONE OF MY MATES FROM
SCHOOL WAS TRICKED!
HE WAS WAITING FOR A BUS
FOR LIKE AN HOUR!

GRAMPS' TIMINGS ARE JUST
A BIT OFF, I THINK.
HE NORMALLY HAS HIS CLUB
ON TUESDAY AND ON SUNDAY.

I THINK IT'S PROBABLY EASY TO MIX THAT UP,
ESPECIALLY IF IT'S SOMETHING YOU'RE LOOKING
FORWARD TO.

HE DID GET IT RIGHT ONCE LAST MONTH.
GOT HIS BUTTONS RIGHT TOO.

THIS DIARY BELONGS TO
SARAH
NO BATH FOR ME

Since we put the cameras in, it's been easier to see how Grandpa's doing and stuff. Make sure he's not wandering off. I can be watching the cameras while eating my breakfast, and you can see him getting frustrated because he's upstairs bound. I can see when Mum tries to give him his breakfast and if he's forgotten how to use a spoon again. Then I can go over if Mum couldn't feed him herself.

The cameras have been really useful for that sort of thing. It's one of those little things that make life easier. Another good trick for when he's having a really bad day or being quite aggressive and not wanting to have his bath, going "no, I'm not having a bath!" is to go upstairs and run the bath!

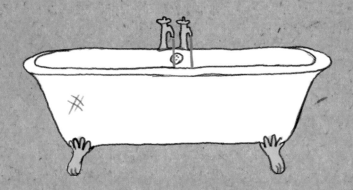

Then, change your shirt, and go back downstairs and say "your bath's ready that you asked for" and then he's quite happy to trot upstairs and have his bath. You just gotta change the goalposts.

If it was a really bad day he would take his clothes off and things. If he didn't have his pants on I'd come back over here and tell Mum and she'd go sort him out.

Then when he'd be fully dressed he'd go and put another pair of pants on. I was quite happy to explain to him that, "you've put another pair of pants on Grandad, we're just going to take them off, then your trousers will feel a bit more comfortable." It's this sort of game that you play.

Except that it keeps happening over and over.

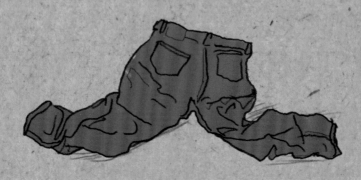

> "Shirt, jumper, shirt, jumper, shirt, jumper, cardigan"

Chapter Four Activities

Loud music!

Turn up some music REALLY LOUD and try to talk over it.
How does it make you feel?
Think of other "alien" rules. For example, would you eat ice-cream for breakfast?

Changes in behaviour

Discuss Gramps' and Grandpa's changes in behaviour as their dementia progresses. What have different family members done to support them?

Draw

Create three pictures to tell the scarecrow story from Grandpa's perspective. Then act out the incident as a play or a radio play.

Technology

Develop a new assistive technology to pitch at Dragon's Den. How would it work? What would it cost? And how could it help someone living with dementia or their families?

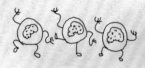

CHAPTER FIVE

"Mr Table Dancer"

Although it can be, dementia's not always a scary thing

MR TABLE DANCER

One of my best memories of Grandpa was last Friday, right after they banned him from golf in the garden! He used to play golf years ago, and for his 85th birthday Mum bought him one of these little garden tees. He was whacking them over the shed so they were ricocheting off the trees hitting next door's window so they had to put a stop to that. Anyway, I decided to go over to cheer him up.

On the bus to school that morning, this one girl at school whose parents are alcoholics turned round and went to me, "Why don't you just tell your Grandpa you don't love him anymore? What's the point? Don't care for him anymore."

I was like, "I can't, I love him." She just didn't understand. People can say, oh it will get better, but it's not going to get better. There's not a cure.

So with that on my mind, I went and got Grandpa some fish and chips and went over his and Gran's house. I knocked on the door and he knew that the white paper meant chips!

I got him to lay the table because it was something that he felt he could do, even though you'd end up with a mixture of cutlery on the table! And he was playing some music, and I went to get something from the front room, and I could hear this tapping...

And when I went back in there, Grandpa was holding on to the chair dancing!

So for the rest of the afternoon we had a bit of a dance and a trot round the room. It was like the old days.

It was so good to see him happy like that.

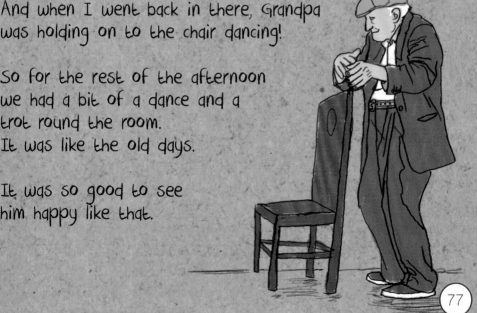

SAM'S DIARY

written by Sam

SWEAR WORDS

I KNOW I SAID NANNY WAS OLD, BUT SHE'S ALSO GOT A MUM WHO'S EVEN OLDER. GRANDNAN.

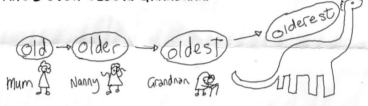

old → older → oldest → olderest

Mum   Nanny   Grandnan

IT'S LIKE SHE'S FROM AN OLD MOVIE, EXCEPT NOT IN BLACK AND WHITE. SHE HASN'T EVEN GOT A TELLY. WE WENT TO VISIT HER YESTERDAY, BUT SHE WAS STILL ASLEEP. I WAS WELL BORED. AND WHEN I GET BORED I ASK QUESTIONS. I ASKED WHY SWEAR WORDS ARE CALLED SWEAR WORDS. MUM SORT OF IGNORED ME, BUT NANNY WANTED TO FIND OUT TOO. SO WE OPENED UP GOOGLE ON MUM'S SAMSUNG GALAXY.

bored bored bored bored bored bored bored bored

im bored!

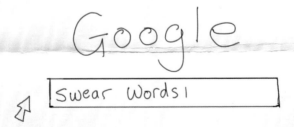

Google

Swear Words!

NANNY SAID THAT IF YOU THINK ABOUT IT, YOU DON'T REALLY KNOW WHY CERTAIN WORDS ARE SWEAR WORDS. I GOT BORED AGAIN WHEN I COULDN'T FIND THE ANSWER, BUT NANNY KEPT GOING.

SAM'S DIARY

written by Sam

SWEAR WORDS

SHE WAS ON THERE FOR LIKE 30 MINUTES LOOKING UP SWEAR WORDS, AND THEN STARTED TESTING THEM ALL OUT AND TELLING US WHAT THEY MEANT.

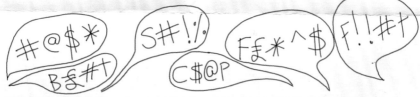

#@$* B&#† S#!% C$@P F£*^$ F!!#†

LIKE THE WORD "CRAP" IS ACTUALLY THE NAME OF THE FELLA WHO INVENTED THE TOILET! BUT FOR SOME REASON THEY STILL WOULDN'T LET ME SAY IT. THEY SAID I WAS TOO YOUNG TO TALK CRAP.

thomas Crapper made me.

THAT WAS JUST BEFORE GRANDNAN WOKE UP. BY THE WAY, SHE SOUNDS LIKE DARTH VADER WHEN SHE SLEEPS! REALLY SCARY. I BET SHE HAS A RED LIGHTSABER AND CAN SHOOT ELECTRICITY FROM HER FINGERS.

AND SHE'S WELL STRICT TOO.

SAM'S DIARY

written by Sam

SWEAR WORDS

SHE WOKE UP AS I WAS SAYING, "CRAP, CRAP, CRAP." I THINK SHE WENT PURPLE.

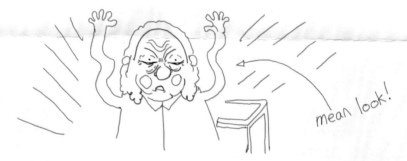

mean look!

SHE SAID, "CHILDREN ARE TO BE SEEN AND NOT HEARD" AND GAVE ME A MEAN LOOK.

NANNY TOLD HER THAT JUST BECAUSE SHE'S OLD, THAT DOESN'T MEAN SHE HAS TO BE GRUMPY.

THAT'S WHY NANNY'S SO GREAT. SHE TREATS ME LIKE I'M A GROWN-UP, AND ALWAYS MAKES ME FEEL LIKE IMPORTANT.

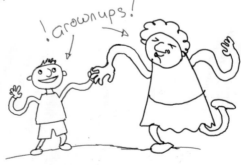

! Grownups!

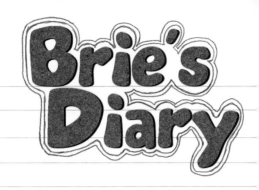

Do you want to know what true love is? It's got nothing to do with Princesses or Magic or One Direction.

True love is my Grannie following my Granddad around the kitchen as he looks for things in drawers. She tries to help him but also tries to put back everything after him. Their whole house is just Grannie trailing after Granddad as he makes a real mess of everything. If he knew that he was doing that, then I'm sure he would have been really, really flabbergasted. Our poor Grannie is a real trooper.

Granddad's become very good at trying to catch or touch something that isn't there.

He keeps saying there's this black lint stuff that he needs to pick up off the floor. And Grannie's always on the floor to help him pick this black stuff up! And she just had two knee replacements! Granddad just spends ages doing it and when we first saw it, we weren't really sure what he was doing, and if we should just leave him or play along.

Grannie would say, "You can't humiliate him. Humour him because it's not his fault." She'd get him to give her all the imaginary black stuff once he'd picked it all up, so she could carry it.

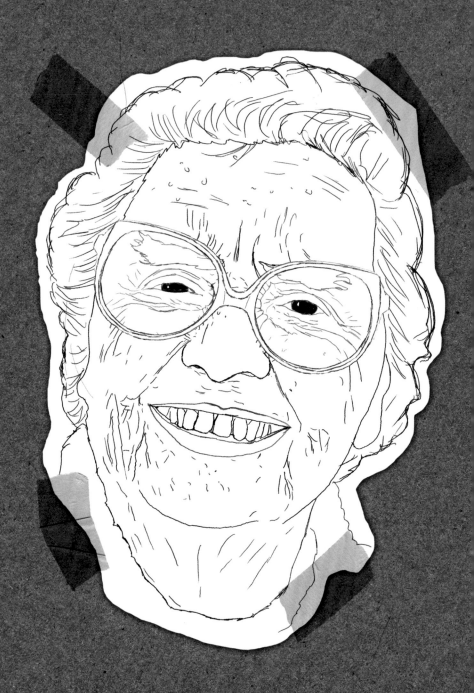

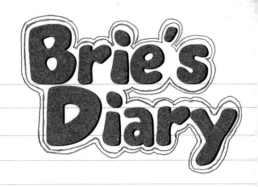

She goes around helping him in these tasks, which of course then validates what he's doing, which is quite nice, I think.

I find it a bit hard, to be honest. I always just look to Grannie for help. You don't really know what to do when someone's seeing something you can't see, or I don't really know what to say because I don't know what they're trying to get at. He's so much older than me, I don't want to make him feel like he's lost his track and I'm trying to prompt him. I really don't know what to do half of the time really!

Grannie just said to play along with it. So I try to follow her lead. She's taught me a lot about how to deal with the Granddad's Dementia.

She has some good rules like:

Make sure that you include him in conversations as much as you can. Just talk to him as if he's there really.

Remember he's there and visibly go over and say hello when you walk into the room. Always introduce yourself.

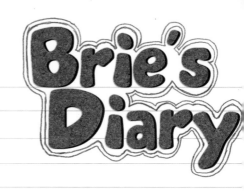

Go along with what he's doing and sort of try to lead him away from it, like if he's emptying all the drawers out, try and help him complete the activity. Then clean up after!

Never ask him a direct question, because if you ask a question, he doesn't know whether he wants a cup of tea, because he can't remember whether he's had a cup of tea this year, this week, yesterday or he doesn't actually know if he even likes tea! You should frame it differently and say, "I'm having a lovely cup of tea now and bringing your tea in." Try and frame everything, especially in the early stages of Dementia. It's the fear and the panic of not knowing stuff that actually makes the person feel worse all the time because it reinforces every minute how not themselves they are.

Play ping pong! Knock a thought or a favourite comfortable conversation to him to see whether he can return it. If he doesn't, then you leave it. But if he returns it, then you can start a conversation on that. Try to find out from him, without asking a question, what he remembers, or what decade the memories might be in, because very often there's more clarity around something that happened 20 or 30 years ago than there is about anything that happened 5 minutes ago.

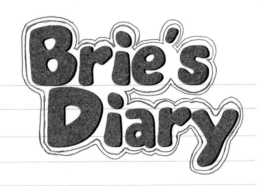

But that's enough Dementia tips for today.

I was trying to tell you about true love, right?

Well, this story will make you believe in it.

As Granddad's Dementia has gotten worse, he sometimes doesn't even recognise Grannie, and he thinks she's the hired help there to sort him out and do things! The other day it became really quite sad because he kept saying she was so rubbish at looking after him, and "Who are you anyway," and "What are your qualifications?" and blah, blah, blah.

And Grannie said, "Just hang on a moment."

So she wandered off and went off in the other room and fetched their wedding photo. Then she came back and gave it to Granddad and said,

"This, this is my qualification!" and then he remembered!

Grannie is amazing.

SARAH

MEMORIES

Gran came up with a great method today! Grandpa's always liked pictures and getting his picture taken, so she pegged up photos of all his children when they were little, and his grandchildren too. And a big family photo with everyone sat in the back garden.
She printed them all out and put everyone's names next to them on a big whiteboard with Velcro.
He would say, "I don't know who you mean, I don't know who you mean!" And you could point to them in the family picture and say, "What's that name say there?" And then with the help, Grandpa would be like, "Oh, I know, I know them." And I think that was quite reassuring for him.

I went to watch, and I was sitting in the corner, and he said, "That girl in the corner, I don't know who she is but she's ever so pretty and she keeps smiling at me." Even though he can't remember who his children are and things, and because I see him so much there's always that little light and that little smile for me.
I'm lucky. Gran's going to show the carers.
Then we can put a time for his lunch and stuff on the board. That'll help, I think...

SAM'S DIARY

written by Sam

NANNY NEWS

NANNY TOLD ME SHE HAS DEMENTIA TODAY.

AND THAT SHE'S HAD IT FOR A WHILE. I GUESS THAT'S
WHY PEOPLE KEPT ASKING ME HOW SHE WAS ALL THE
TIME. I WOULD ALWAYS SAY SHE'S AS SILLY AS EVER,
AND THEY'D GIVE ME A VERY SAD LOOK.
IT WAS ALWAYS A BIT A STRANGE. IT'S FUNNY BECAUSE
SHE'S ALWAYS BEEN THE SAME TO ME. ALWAYS FULL
OF LAUGHTER. SHE SAYS THAT'S THE BEST WAY TO BE!
WHATEVER DEMENTIA IS, IT'S NOT HER.

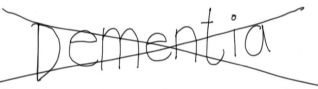

SHE'S ALWAYS GOING TO BE MY NANNY. IT DOESN'T
CHANGE HER. AND IF SHE LOSES MORE BRAIN CELLS,
WELL, WE'LL ALL BE THERE WITH HER DOING THAT
TOGETHER, AND IF THAT MEANS WE CAN HAVE A GIGGLE
AND A BOOGIE ON THE WAY TOO, THEN I THINK THAT'S
THE BEST THING TO DO.

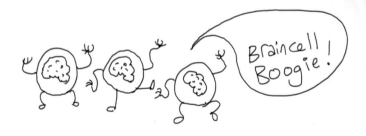

SAM'S DIARY

written by Sam

NANNY NEWS

MUM'S ORGANISED IT SO I CAN LEARN TO HELP CARE FOR NANNY AND GO TO CARERS SUPPORT GROUPS AND MEET OTHER KIDS WHO HAVE GRANDPARENTS WITH DEMENTIA TOO. IT'S LIKE A KIND OF A FAMILY THING REALLY. I EVEN FOUND OUT THAT A FEW OF MY FRIENDS AT SCHOOL HAD GRANDPARENTS WITH DEMENTIA TOO! NANNY HAD SOME GOOD ADVICE. SHE SAID,

"RIGHT, YOU'VE GOT THIS TIME NOW, DON'T DWELL ON IT, DON'T TAKE IT SO SERIOUSLY, AND IT'S NOT THE END OF THE BOOK, IT'S JUST THE BEGINNING OF THE NEXT CHAPTER."

AND ANY BOOK WITH MY NANNY IN IT SOUNDS LIKE A PRETTY GOOD BOOK TO ME!

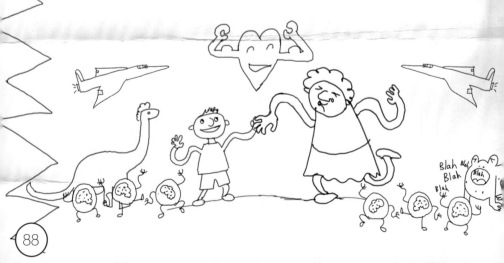

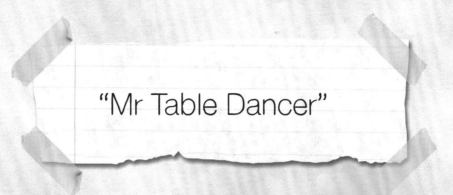

"Mr Table Dancer"

Chapter Five Activities

Blog

Imagine you are Sarah and you have started writing a blog about dementia. One of your friends says, "My grandad doesn't speak to me. He just looks bored all of the time, but I don't know what to say to him." How will you respond?

Family tree

Create your own family and friends tree using photos. Label the photos and perhaps include people's favourite hobbies, food or music.

Record a vlog

Record a YouTube video about how best to talk to and support someone living with dementia. Dramatise one of Grannie's rules.

Research

Who is the oldest person you know? Find some music from when they were a child and play it to them. See what they think.

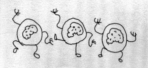

CHAPTER SIX

"The Christmas decision"

Thinking about the future

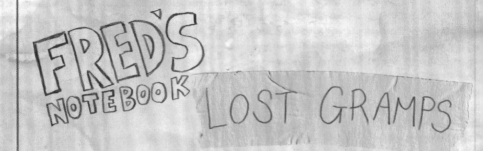

FRED'S NOTEBOOK
LOST GRAMPS

MUM SAID I MIGHT BE GETTING MY ROOM BACK SOON.
THAT MAKES ME SAD. IT'S GRAMPS' ROOM NOW.
BESIDES, WHO ELSE WOULD MESS WITH SIMON,
ESPECIALLY WHEN HE BRINGS HIS GIRLFRIEND ROUND?!
BUT MAYBE MUM'S RIGHT...

GRAMPS IS GETTING WORSE EVERY DAY.
HE'S NOT REALLY TALKING MUCH, AND HE'S ALWAYS
GETTING HIMSELF LOST. HE'S NOT BEEN GOING TO
THE CLUB MUCH EITHER. I GET LOST SOMETIMES AT
SCHOOL, AND I THINK IT MUST BE A BIT LIKE THAT.
IT'S LIKE YOU KNOW WHERE EVERYTHING IS SUPPOSED
TO BE. BUT THEN WHEN YOU TURN UP IT'S NOT THERE...
A BIT LIKE MY MATHS CLASS.

ANYWAY, LAST NIGHT GRAMPS
CAME DOWN AND MUM SAID,
"WHERE ARE YOU GOING?" AND
HE SAID, "TO THE BATHROOM."
THEN HE JUST WALKED INTO THE
LOUNGE AND I WAS LIKE,
"YOU'VE FOUND US INSTEAD!"
THAT REALLY CONFUSED HIM, I THINK.

HE WAS ALL LIKE, "I KNOW THAT!" SO HE WENT BACK UPSTAIRS. NEXT THING WE KNOW HE WAS PEEING INTO A PLASTIC BOX IN HIS ROOM, BECAUSE HE COULDN'T FIND THE BATHROOM. AND THE BATHROOM IS RIGHT NEXT DOOR! IT WAS PRETTY GROSS!

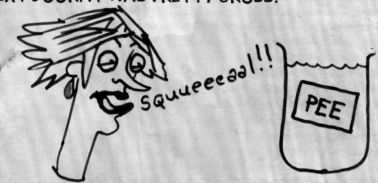

I ASKED SIMON'S GIRLFRIEND IF SHE WANTED TO SEE IT. SHE SQUEALED A LITTLE BIT AND SIMON PUNCHED ME IN THE ARM. IT WAS WORTH IT.

I DON'T WANT GRAMPS TO GO AWAY THOUGH. HE'S OUR GRAMPS. I THINK IT'S A TOUGH DECISION FOR MUM AND DAD. THEY'RE REALLY WORRIED ABOUT HIM. MUM SAYS WE COULD STILL VISIT HIM, AND THAT THERE WILL BE PEOPLE AT THIS HOME THAT CAN LOOK AFTER HIM BETTER. I DON'T KNOW WHAT'S SO HARD ABOUT LOOKING AFTER HIM. JUST GIVE HIM SOME WAR MOVIES AND A CROSSWORD AND HE'S FINE.

I DON'T WANT MY ROOM BACK.

I WANT MY GRAMPS BACK.

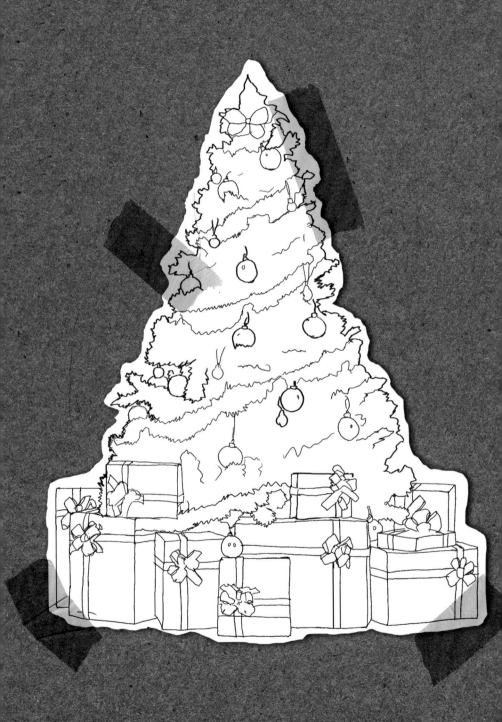

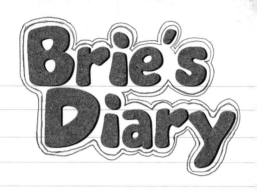

It's almost New Year, and I'm still not feeling so good.

The day after Boxing day, Mum and Dad decided that Granddad should go into a care home. Granddad had a really bad decline over the holiday. It was that fast from being here and being a bit vague, to not being here. I don't really remember the transition time between how I remember him as the Granddad who tells me everything I could possibly want to know about anything, to the Granddad who couldn't really talk to me properly.

On Christmas, he did raise his eyebrows at me in the kind of hmmm expression about whatever I was saying about my random day, so he was still him then. It felt like he knew that I was there, but even if it was only for a short bit, it did make me feel that maybe some of the time he can hear me. Grannie says that he sometimes makes a few noises and one time he even said Mary's name. Mary used to get the best responses out of Granddad. I don't know why - she just mastered the art of speech, or something that really triggers his memories maybe.

I think he did say hello to me once, and hello to Mary. I think he almost even managed to get out a few words to Mary before, but otherwise she's the one who had the best success with him.

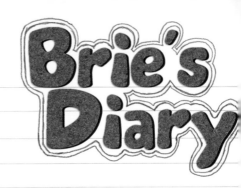

Then during Christmas dinner, it was quite difficult because he kept
thinking something was dropping off the table but there wasn't
anything there and he was quite shaky. And then when we
did the presents, the wrapping paper would get in the way.
He would try and pick it up but then it would get quite hard
because of his co-ordination.

After dinner, Grannie said that they should head home. But simple
things like trying to get on a jacket were like 10 times harder than
you'd imagine. Then we had to keep taking him away from the car so
we could re-approach the car to try and work out how to get in the
car because he lost the ability.

I remember that night our phone was off the hook by mistake.
Someone had obviously knocked it over when we were unwrapping the
presents. Grannie had been trying to get through on the line because
Granddad just wouldn't go to bed, and he was just standing there.
I don't know what he was doing just standing there, he just wouldn't
come to bed. Grannie tried everything, but in the end she had to call
an ambulance. . . because he took all his clothes off. . .
and just stood there naked.

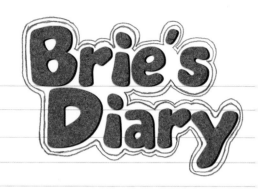

When they got to the hospital, Gran said that she had to wheelchair him backwards around the entire hospital.

She just couldn't make it go forwards, as it was broken or something. So she pulled it backwards through the whole hospital, and then she got it stuck in a doorway! Grannie nearly put her hip out pulling Granddad through, never mind those knees of hers! We were quite worried in the morning because we just woke up and obviously it's a bit bad with all the phones being off the hook.

It was the one night where she really needed some help. That's when Mum and Dad made the decision... when Grannie couldn't get him into bed, she couldn't cope any more. They decided before Grannie manages to get all the things in... like a bed at her house for him with the sides. I think that's when Grannie realised she really does need to have him in a home just for a bit, because she was running out of sleep really.

She's been up most of the night for the last couple of weeks, and she couldn't really carry on like that. Mum says that at least until she's got the proper carers scheduled to come round, and have the right environment for him at home, he needs to be away.

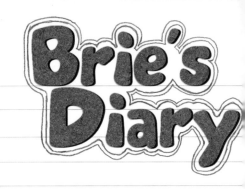

I guess when it gets to this point, it's about thinking through all the possible changes that might happen based on the research that's out there, and then thinking ahead to, well,

"What would my options be if that person that I love changes in this way or that way or the other way?"

SARAH

NOT HIMSELF

Grandpa's in a care home now. We got to the stage where we were finding we couldn't cope with him at home anymore. He became too aggressive. You could tell by his eyes. There was a kind of blankness in the eyes and you knew that you needed to be the door side that day because he could be laughing in your face one minute and the next minute... He was treating us like the scarecrow in the field.

So, yeah. It was a good idea. He's not been doing "well" there, I don't think. It's like he's gone back to childhood in, like, his food needs to be cut up for him, or mashed up for him and he's completely chair-bound.

He would never eat a curry or anything, it wasn't him. He was a roast sort of person and they put meals in front of him and one day the nurse said, "Oh, he hasn't eaten his curry today".

99

It was all colours, colourful rice, colours, Grandpa loved colours and the alternative was shepherds pie, dull boring shepherds pie. He'd just turned round and went, "I want that one", and so they'd put the curry in front of him and he forgotten how to eat it. So he was just looking at it. He wouldn't drink either. But we had a trick for that at least.

We used to take him out and we'd get him a pint, a shandy, or a Guinness, and we'd sit there and go, "Cheers, down the hatch!" And that would go down. Although sometimes he liked to pour his Guinness over his roast dinner...

But in the care home, we'd say, "Here's your glass. Cheers, down the hatch", and he would drink water like he was drinking a pint, and you could get him to down 4 glasses. That sort of thing really works wonders.

He's been sharing a room. The man in the other bed kept saying that Grandpa was stealing things from him and they kept finding them in my Grandpa's locker, but it couldn't be Grandpa because Grandpa can't walk.

And then one night after they put him to bed, one of the staff sat in the dark in the room to see what was going on, because they kept finding stuff in Grandpa's locker. Grandpa would sit upright, swing his legs out the bed, walk across the room, raid this old boy's locker, calling him all the names under the sun, and then put all the stuff in his locker and then go back to bed.

I guess he's just not himself anymore.

I was there today to help him write some Christmas cards. It was like giving a toddler a pen. He just scribbled on the page and I kept writing Grandpa on a piece of paper because he kept going to me, "How do you spell it again, how do you spell it again?"

So I'd write it down for him again and then he could get the G... and then the rest of it was a sort of squiggle. It's so sad.

He could write so beautifully before. That's what he did. But I was happy I got to do this with him.

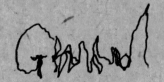

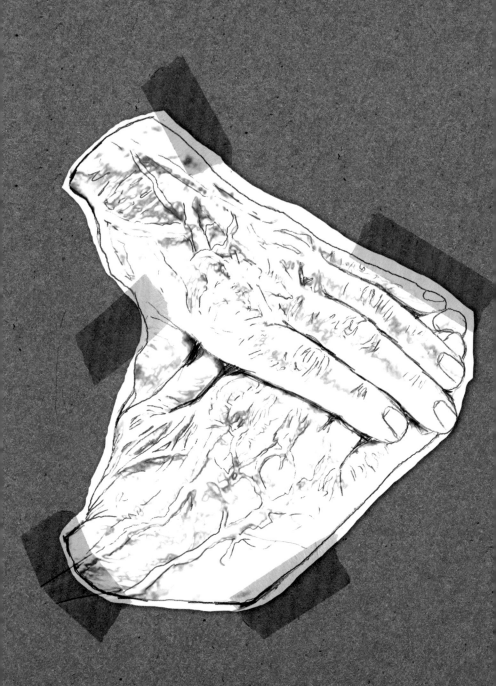

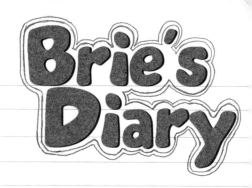

Brie's Diary

This is hard to write. He's very thin.
He's really thin. He's really very thin.

I saw Granddad today at the home. I was really surprised at how much he changed because I hadn't seen him for at least a few weeks, but in those few weeks he went from being able to put on his own coat to not even walking and talking. I actually couldn't believe that so much could change in such a short time. Mary didn't want to come. She was all, "I don't want to see him if he's declined to that point. I want to remember him the way he was."

I really had no idea he would be that bad when I went in, Mum had said that he was worse now that he's in the care home.

But he was quite a lot worse. He couldn't talk at all, he barely made noises. Just sat there shaking and jerking unfortunately.

Grannie's here from 7 in the morning until 10 at night, every single day, and she's been caring for him, helping him eat. He gets cleaned up at the beginning and end of the day by a care company that come in. They have a hoist that they use to get him in and out of the bed.

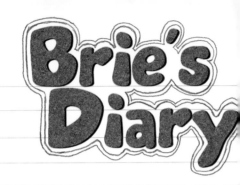

If he got a major chest infection or something, he'd get pneumonia and die probably but I don't know really. He eats by reflex, Grannie puts some food in his mouth, but it's like having a baby or a small toddler. She's so good with him it's just□ she's incredible.
Some of the other residents even think she's a member of staff!
I don't think I'm really equipped for this.

I wish it was the kind of the disease where when he got to the point where you were like, "That's it, he's gone," and then it would all end there. Why would he have to keep going like this? I know it's different for every family. Granddad wasn't hugely loud, violent, abusive or any of those things which I know can be a side effect. I mean he was strict, but like in a good way. I think that's partly because he's a Pharmacist. He knew in time what the prognosis was and maybe he was self controlled about it.

Who knows what's going on, but I know its been a very very difficult journey and there isn't a one size fits all. And things can change quite quickly and dramatically.

I just want people to enjoy the time they have with them.
It's a scary thing.

SARAH

WHAT i LEARNT FROM GRANDPA

Grandpa passed away the end of December and was in a care home for the last eight weeks of his life. I miss him. But I think he's in a better place now. They say Alzheimer's affects people in really different ways. I think I'm going to study it now. I want to help people like Grandpa.

At my job at the shop, we had a lady come in and you could tell she had Alzheimer's, and her husband was trying to get her to buy a hat, but she didn't want it. The husband kept saying, "You look lovely in it, you look lovely in it." And she's going, "No I don't, no I don't!" really angrily. Then she wanted a mirror.

So I got her a mirror, and her husband was holding it for her and again she said, "No! You're holding it wrong."

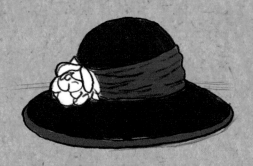

But learning from Grandpa, sometimes just a different face changes everything. I asked if I could hold the mirror and the lady kept asking, "Do I look alright? Do I look alright?" She was really self-conscious because she didn't know herself. I told her she did. Then she decided, "Ah yes, it does look quite nice." And then she was quite happy with the whole setup of things. She didn't even want to take it off! I remember her husband's smile.

That was a look of relief.

It was a bit like Grandpa with his second pair of trousers. You can't change that person, you've got to learn to adapt yourself. It's talking to them in a different way like, "I'm going to put this on you now." And you do it in a fun way, not in a depressing way. There's no point saying, "You can't do it like that" or "Stand like this", but if you let them think they're doing it their own way, it's so much easier.

Alzheimer's or Dementia makes you see people in a different light.

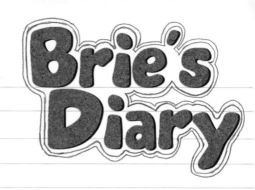

Brie's Diary

Grannie called today. It was good news.

They're going to let Granddad come home! He's much more stable now, they said. It must be really tough to work there at the care home. You have to look after so many people, and none of them will ever remember you.

I think it's a good thing Grannie's been with him, nursing him and giving him the one-to-one attention he needs. She's even been shaving his beard and washing his hair and putting on his favourite aftershave. He's probably the smartest-looking guy in the place! But they really do need to be taken care of so much. And I guess there's only so much the carers can do in a day, aftershave on every guest might be a bit much! Grannie's making them look bad! ;-)

Anyway, we've been down at Grannie and Granddad's getting it all sorted for him so they can tick the box and let him come back. Grannie's going to be so much more relaxed when she can take care of him from home. We put in an electric bed in the lounge with sides to stop Granddad falling out. And then there's his padded wheelchair, and the hoist, like they have at the care home. It's all kitted out. The lounge kind of looks like a hospital now.

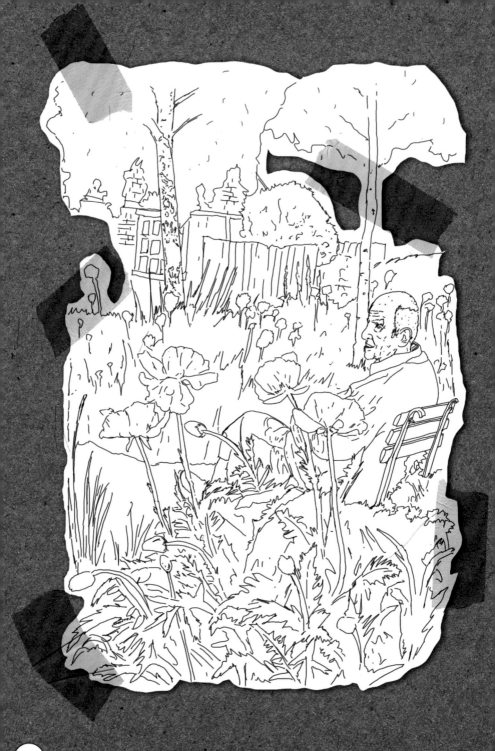

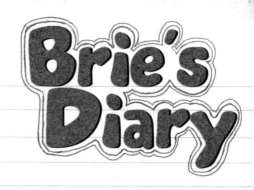

I'm really glad Mary changed her mind about not wanting to see Granddad. She's been studying Dementia and getting involved with organisations like Alzheimer's Research and she knows what needs to go where. She says that she felt so helpless, because there's no cure. So doing something practical helps!

Grannie's going to be able to roll Granddad into the garden really easily when the weather's good. He's always loved that garden. Listening to his jazz while gardening as Grannie reads a book. It's so nice that they can keep doing that together. Granddad can sit outside and they can just be together in their garden. It sounds really peaceful and relaxed. Which is just what they need, I think, especially now that he's so close to the end. He's still able to eat by reflex and sometimes he raises an eyebrow or smiles which is nice. We'll still be able to visit him and talk about random stuff, and maybe that cat will visit too!

But now that he's coming home, I can just see him sitting in that garden, with his eyes closed, bathed in a ray of sunlight.
Like an old leaf getting ready to fall from the tree.

And he's smiling.

Chapter Six Activities

Blog

Write a blog about what you have learned about dementia.

Design a care home

If you could build any care home you can imagine, what would you do to help people living with dementia?

Roleplay

Put yourself into the shoes of Fred. How does he feel about Gramps possibly moving into a care home?

Now put yourself into the shoes of Brie. Did she think it was the right decision for Granddad to move into a care home? Would other members of her family think differently? Think about the reasons for and against it.

Home adaptations

What adaptations can be made to make it easier to live at home? Draw a room with some of the things that may need to be adapted.

Care

Do further research into how care is funded. Do families get financial support to help pay for a loved one in a care home or living at home?

Share

Think about what you have learned from this book. Write a review and share it with us on Facebook.

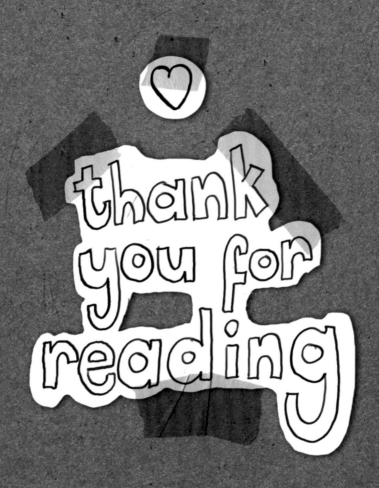

WHAT IS DEMENTIA?

Dementia is a term that is used to describe a collection of symptoms including memory loss, problems with reasoning and communication skills, and a reduction in a person's abilities and skills in carrying out daily tasks such as washing, dressing, cooking and caring for self.

There are a number of different types of dementia, the most common being Alzheimer's disease, vascular dementia, frontal temporal dementia and dementia with Lewy bodies.

Some people are diagnosed as having mixed dementia; this is when the presentation shows the person to have elements of more than one type of dementia.

Dementia is a progressive condition, which means the symptoms will gradually get worse. This progression will vary from person to person and each person will experience dementia in a different way.

Source: Dementia UK

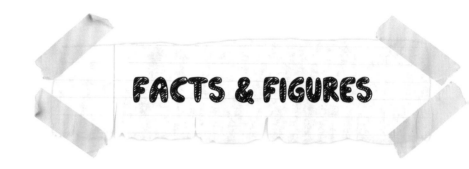

FACTS & FIGURES

Alzheimer's disease is the most common type of dementia, affecting 62 per cent of those diagnosed.

Other types of dementia include vascular dementia which affects 17 per cent of those diagnosed and mixed dementia which affects 10 per cent of those diagnosed.

There are an estimated **35.6 MILLION** people living with dementia and the numbers affected will double every 20 years, rising to **115.4 MILLION** in 2050.

Another **7.7 MILLION PEOPLE** will develop dementia around the world every year.

There is no cure for Alzheimer's disease or any other type of dementia. Delaying the onset of dementia by five years would halve the number of deaths from the condition, saving 30,000 lives a year.

Facts: Alzheimer's Society

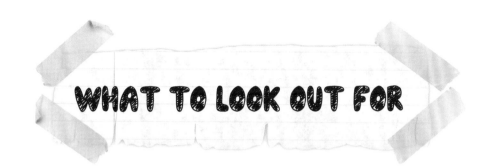

WHAT TO LOOK OUT FOR

LOSS OF MEMORY

This particularly affects short-term memory – for example, forgetting what happened earlier in the day, not being able to recall conversations, being repetitive or forgetting the way home from the shops.
Long-term memory is usually still quite good.

PROBLEMS WITH COMMUNICATION

Some people experience problems with expressing themselves, talking and understanding things. They get confused about words and might use the wrong words for common things and mix words up. Reading and understanding written text can become problematic.

MOOD CHANGES

People with dementia may be withdrawn, sad, frightened or angry about what is happening to them.

Although the person will have some of the above symptoms, the degree to which they affect an individual will vary and not all people will have all of these symptoms.

Source: Dementia UK

WORD SEARCH

Dementia may affect:

Memory

Communication

Personal hygiene

Orientation

Emotions

Judgement

Behaviour

Reasoning

Mobility

Basic Skills

```
            C  S O U D D U O R E
         T E O U T N Q I  I T B N A M R
      S E R  L  A M F A ⊦ C T Q P ⌐ C N A  M L
      T C  A G A V B S Y ⌐ P N E M O T I O N S
    C V E K ⌐ R X ⌐ ⌐ D P  R T O J R Z M A B  B N T H
   H T N I E T T Z J F  B O G V X S N M E ⌐  I M H M A
   I N N E A S J U D G E M E N T O Q U I T L E ⋃ E T ⌐
  E M A A ⌐ I N J T R R H E I T O N U N E N I I I S A A N
  I ⌐ E M A E M E N E K A M A ⌐ N A I I E ⊢ T A Y ⌐ O T D
  I J N E D W T S T  ⋃ A N V B R A C ⌐ V C Y K Y I ⋃ D ⌐ A D
  H T A ⌐ ⌐ B A S I C S K I ⌐ ⌐ S U H I A A E S S S H R S I T
  V A N N Y E N O C A O ⌐ ⌐ O ⌐ I M P Y Q T J D E ⌐ T T M E W
   Z S W Q E I N K W N T ⋃ O I R E G M I I A E ⌐ ⌐ ⋃ N Y T
   X ⌐ Y O E O R A I Q R ⌐ ⌐ T N I ⋃ O ⋃ I ⌐ E A M G O
      P H N I ⌐ N E ⋃ ⋃ B A Y E X N A D S ⋃ Y X 6 T
         G E ⅃ N A E B N O ⌐ I D X I T M D ⌐
               ⌐ N E O ⋃ T Z B A H Z T
               ⌐ V E N ⌐ O R O T N
               A D M T ⋃ C J
                 B E Z ⋃ X
                 N E N N
                 R A ⌐ S
                 S T E S
                   E J ⌐
                   O ⋃ E
                   A R T
```

Can you find them all?

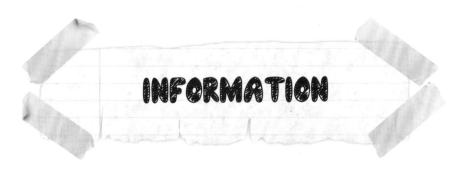

INFORMATION

If someone in your family is living with dementia or you suspect they might have dementia, here are some great resources that might help.

And remember, this is not anybody's fault, and you are not alone.

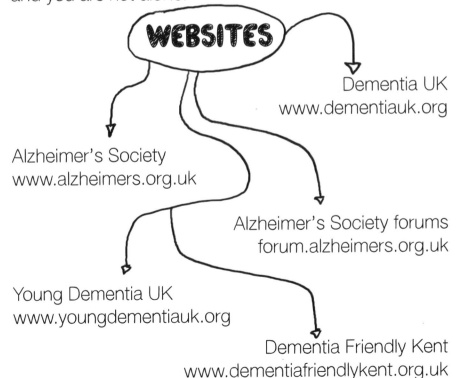

WEBSITES

Dementia UK
www.dementiauk.org

Alzheimer's Society
www.alzheimers.org.uk

Alzheimer's Society forums
forum.alzheimers.org.uk

Young Dementia UK
www.youngdementiauk.org

Dementia Friendly Kent
www.dementiafriendlykent.org.uk

SUPPORT

If you are a dementia carer and need more information or support, these sites are a great place to find them.

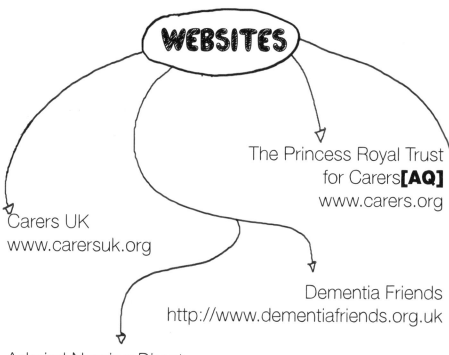

WEBSITES

The Princess Royal Trust for Carers**[AQ]**
www.carers.org

Carers UK
www.carersuk.org

Dementia Friends
http://www.dementiafriends.org.uk

Admiral Nursing Direct
www.dementiauk.org/what-we-do/admiral-nursing-direct

Dementia Alliance International
www.dementiaallianceinternational.org

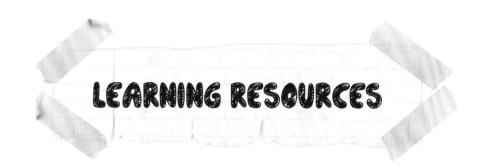

LEARNING RESOURCES

Additional educational content and Learning Resource by:

NICKI KOMOROWSKI

Nicki is an educational writer, photographer and a secondary school teacher with almost twenty years of classroom experience. She is an English, Media and Film specialist and has written a wide variety of teaching resources.

The Dementia Diaries project has grown to include a Learning Resource pack which is curriculum-ready for a classroom, community learning or home education setting.

The Learning Resource pack has been produced using the Dementia Diaries as source material for lessons, games and educational experiences by qualified teachers and carers. The Learning Resource pack was designed by the same team behind the Dementia Diaries. The Learning Resource pack has been targeted at KS2 and KS3. There are no right or wrong answers.

CONNECT WITH OTHERS

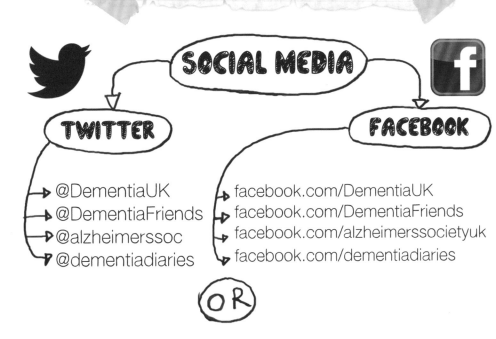

SOCIAL MEDIA

TWITTER

→ @DementiaUK
→ @DementiaFriends
→ @alzheimerssoc
→ @dementiadiaries

FACEBOOK

→ facebook.com/DementiaUK
→ facebook.com/DementiaFriends
→ facebook.com/alzheimerssocietyuk
→ facebook.com/dementiadiaries

OR

DISCOVER THE DEMENTIA DIARIES
LEARNING RESOURCES HERE

SCAN ME

Or visit
facebook.com/
dementiadiaries
to join the
conversation

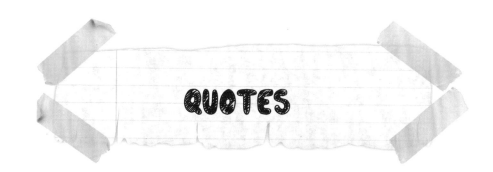

A beautiful book from the first page to the last word.
Anne Child MBE

The work you are doing is so moving and so very important.
Artz Philadelphia

WOW... A 'must' for all those families who find themselves having to have that awkward conversation with the kids about what is happening around them. It really puts things into perspective. Well done.
Amazon review

Whenever you want to change how a community thinks about conditions like this you always start with children. For two reasons; first of all children go straight to the heart of any issue, they are not polite, they are extremely honest and they have a way of connecting straight-away to the problem.
Trudy Dean, Chair of Select Committee

Absolutely brilliant book. Well written and great to share together as a family. Helps get those conversations going. Highly recommend this book :-)
Amazon Review

The resources are fun and engaging. My students loved getting to know the characters, both young and old, in more depth and they were really able to empathise with those living with Dementia and their families.
Teacher – Lisa Herron, Rochester Independent College

I work within a Home Treatment Service that specialise in supporting those with a diagnosis or probable diagnosis. I have the belief publications like this could well aid in reducing stigma attached to a diagnosis of dementia. Not only can it bring some comfort to those with a new or long standing diagnosis and to their families/carers, but it can also provide education.
Jennifer Cooper, Mental Health Nurse, Sittingbourne

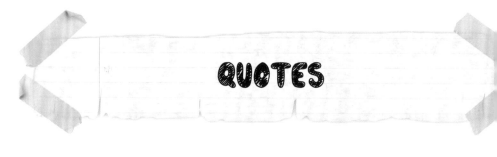

QUOTES

Once I started to read "The Dementia Diaries" I couldn't put it down, & I'm not a reader. Some parts of the book I found quite humorous, other parts reduced me to tears. The attitude of these young people to dementia is very uplifting. As a fairly new carer I can learn. An exceptional book – very well done to all who contributed. Thank you.
Jean W, Carer

We need innovative resources, such as the Dementia Diaries as an educational resource for everyone. This novel in cartoons will engage children and adults around the world. In fact, the idea of making a book about dementia by children is ground-breaking. I highly recommend the Dementia Diaries to anyone that wants to learn about the challenges of dementia through the eyes of young children.
Sophie Okolo, Aging Professional, USA

This is not only a book about Dementia. It is also a book about the wisdom of children and young people. First of all, perhaps, it is a book about the surprising depths of love between generations. Written by young people who have the courage to face the brutal facts of life. It is carefully leading you by the hand into new perceptions and discoveries of one of the diseases that we all fear. I have a sister who is now in the final stage of Alzheimer's, and the book has made me laugh and giggle with her over and over again. Read this book – now. And share it – as soon as you can.
Jens Peter Jensen, Social Innovation Platforms Denmark

A WORD FROM THE CONTRIBUTORS

Brian, Contributor

I was just blown away as far as seeing the book. I thought this is great, this is just the right thing for children to read. The book is something children will readily read with ease.

Tom, Contributor

If we can educate our youngsters and it becomes the norm and everyone learns about it in our schools, we will have a whole generation growing up without the stigma that surrounds dementia.

Alison, Contributor

Through telling our story in the character of Brie in *The Dementia Diaries*, we would like to raise awareness about dementia which we hope, in turn, will lead to more funding for research to find causes and cures. We know that our Granddad, who used to be a pharmacist, would have wanted us to talk about what happened and how wonderfully our Grannie looked after him as well as our own experiences of his dementia. We hope that this book will be a comfort to other young people who have dementia in their family.

Jack, Contributor

We came up with an idea for the book which was easy to understand and what would make it clearer what dementia was and why people got it and what people were going through. I am really pleased how it came out, it was just how I imagined it to be.

Jasmine, Contributor

It's just a book of everything that's comes together and it's a book of everything, all my memories of him and it's really going to help other people.

Imogen, Contributor

It tells people about dementia and it can help them through their dementia in the family.

Raisa, Contributor

Sharing my story, I now feel more open about living with someone with dementia and its not a big hush hush. I feel it should be shared now, not kept to yourself.

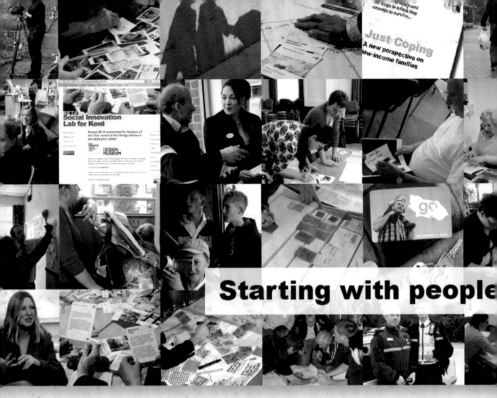

Starting with people

THE SOCIAL INNOVATION LAB FOR KENT (S.I.L.K.)

SILK was set up in 2007 with two ambitions. First, to provide a creative environment for a wide range of people to work together on some of the toughest challenges the county faces. And second, by drawing upon best practice from business, design, social science and community development, as well as our own experiences here in Kent, SILK set out to establish a collaborative way of working that places people at its heart. Emma Barrett Palmer has been directing the SILK programme since 2009.

www.socialinnovation.typepad.com/silk/
@SILKteam

124